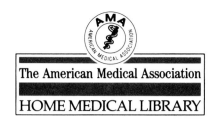

The American Medical Association

HOME MEDICAL LIBRARY

# EXERCISE, FITNESS, AND HEALTH

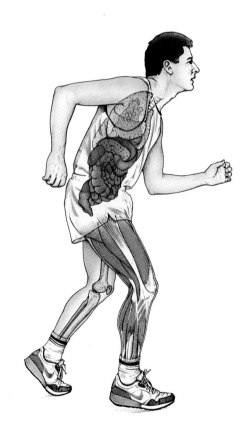

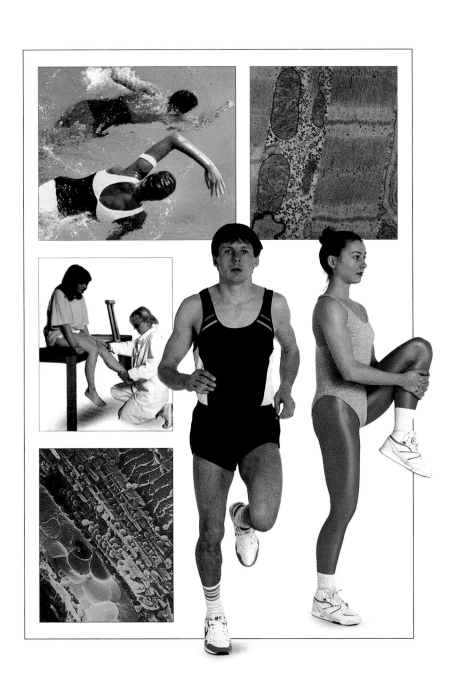

# THE AMERICAN MEDICAL ASSOCIATION

# EXERCISE, FITNESS, AND HEALTH

Medical Editor
CHARLES B. CLAYMAN, MD

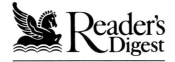

THE READER'S DIGEST ASSOCIATION, INC.
Pleasantville, New York/Montreal

The information in this book reflects current medical knowledge. The
recommendations and information are appropriate in most cases;
however, they are not a substitute for medical diagnosis. For specific
information concerning your personal medical condition, the AMA
suggests that you consult a physician.

The names of organizations, products, or alternative therapies appearing
in this book are given for informational purposes only. Their inclusion
does not imply AMA endorsement, nor does the omission of any
organization, product, or alternative therapy indicate AMA disapproval.

The AMA Home Medical Library is distinct from and unrelated to the
series of health books published by Random House, Inc., in conjunction
with the American Medical Association under the names ''The AMA Home
Reference Library'' and ''The AMA Home Health Library.''

**Library of Congress Cataloging in Publication Data**

Exercise, fitness, and health/medical editor, Charles B. Clayman.
     p.  cm. — (The American Medical Association home medical
library)
  At head of title: The American Medical Association.
  Includes index.
  ISBN 0-89577-373-2
  1. Exercise. 2. Physical fitness. 3. Sports — Accidents and
injuries — Prevention. I. Clayman, Charles B. II. American Medical
Association. III. Series.
RA781.E893 1991
613.7 — dc20

                                                90-44523

# FOREWORD

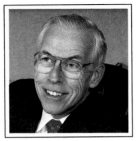

Exercising regularly to keep yourself physically fit is a vital part of a healthy life. In recent years, many Americans have incorporated exercise into their routine and have greatly improved their mental and physical health as a result. This volume of the AMA Home Medical Library is designed to make clear that exercise is important for virtually everyone, not just for professional athletes. We as doctors share your concern for, and interest in, physical fitness as one vital element in your wellness program. This volume gives you practical information you can use to get in shape and stay in shape, with specific guidelines for all members of your family.

The old theory that exercise must be strenuous to benefit your health may have led to overexertion and injury in the past, and undoubtedly served to discourage many people from trying to exercise. However, recent research has confirmed that even moderate exercise performed regularly helps protect us from disease and prolong life expectancy.

Of course, physical activity carries a risk of injury, but most of the injuries are minor strains or sprains. To help you deal with and prevent accidents, we have included information on various sports injuries around the body, indicating symptoms and some likely causes. This volume also offers practical advice on the process of recovery, including first-aid measures for the first 48 hours after injury, practical advice on when to see your doctor, and an illustrated guide to rehabilitation exercises that you might find helpful.

We at the American Medical Association hope that you and your family enjoy your exercise and that it leads to improvements in your health and general well-being.

**JAMES S. TODD, MD**
Executive Vice President
American Medical Association

# CONTENTS

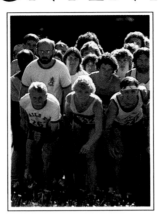

Foreword    5

## CHAPTER ONE

## EXERCISE: A HEALTHY HABIT    8

## CHAPTER TWO

## EXERCISE IS FOR EVERYONE    38

## CHAPTER THREE

## A GUIDE TO FITNESS    56

## CHAPTER FOUR

## HOW TO EXERCISE SAFELY    66

## CHAPTER FIVE

## SPORTS INJURIES AROUND THE BODY    84

## CHAPTER SIX

## RECOVERING FROM AN INJURY    116

A-Z of Drugs in Sports 136    Index of Sports Injuries 140

Index    142

# CHAPTER ONE

# EXERCISE: A HEALTHY HABIT

INTRODUCTION

THE NEED FOR PHYSICAL ACTIVITY

HOW EXERCISE AFFECTS YOUR BODY

THE BENEFITS OF EXERCISE

TYPES OF EXERCISE

CHOOSING YOUR EXERCISE

EXERCISE AND DIET

ALTHOUGH MOST PEOPLE are aware that exercise is good for their health, for many people the most strenuous exercise they get is climbing a flight of stairs at the end of the day. The list of excuses people give for not exercising is seemingly endless. They say they are not athletically inclined, that work takes up all their time, that they are always too tired, or that they are too overweight or out of condition. In fact, exercise is accessible to everyone, it need not take much time, and it is of great benefit in banishing fatigue and in helping you to lose weight.

Today's medical thinking stresses that the elderly benefit from regular exercise, too. If you continue to stay active throughout your life, there is evidence that you are more likely to live longer and stay in good health, although eventually you may not be able

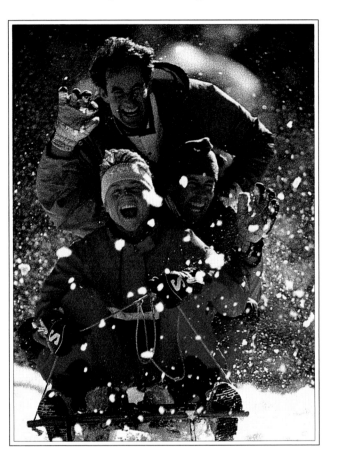

to push yourself as much as you once did. An ever-increasing number of people are involved in some form of regular physical activity or are participating in sports during their leisure time. Hundreds of thousands of people jog or take walks at least once a week, either to stay in shape or just for the fun of it. Many take part in sponsored walks or runs.

This opening chapter describes the physiological changes that occur in your body during exercise, explains how regular exercise improves the efficiency and performance of organs such as your heart, lungs, and muscles, and describes the many short- and long-term benefits that come from exercising regularly. The body gains the energy it needs for exercise from several chemical processes. This chapter discusses the important difference between aerobic and anaerobic exercises and how they affect your body. The main types of exercise are described, with examples of aerobic activities, strength training, and flexibility routines. There are many exercises from which to choose. Some people prefer to exercise in the privacy of their homes, while others stay motivated only if they exercise in a group. A regular workout in a gym, or using exercise equipment in a health club, has become a regular activity for many people. However, you do not need expensive equipment in order to exercise.

This chapter concludes with a discussion of diet, exercise, and fitness. We dispel some myths about dietary aids and we offer some useful tips on the best food to eat before exercising and how much fluid your body needs during exercise.

# THE NEED FOR PHYSICAL ACTIVITY

The ancient philosophers recognized the importance of exercise in terms of general health. In recent years there has been a renewed interest in, and emphasis on, physical exercise. For most of human history, only a small percentage of people in each generation were able to play games and sports. Most people had to work hard physically to earn a living and found the working day tiring enough. Any leisure time they had was spent resting and relaxing. As recently as the early years of this century, most occupations and routine tasks at home still required plenty of physical activity. But labor-saving machinery was gradually introduced and, by the 1950s, factories, farms, transportation, and even the family home were being mechanized.

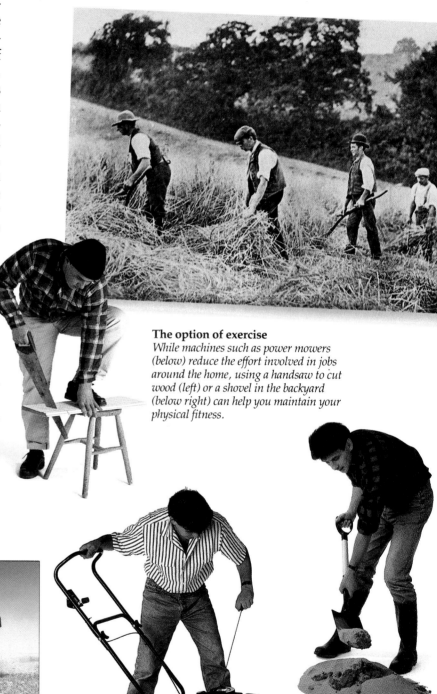

**The option of exercise**
*While machines such as power mowers (below) reduce the effort involved in jobs around the home, using a handsaw to cut wood (left) or a shovel in the backyard (below right) can help you maintain your physical fitness.*

**Changes in farming**
*While countless agricultural workers once tilled, planted, weeded, and harvested the land (top left and right), that work is now being carried out by a smaller work force operating agricultural machinery (below).*

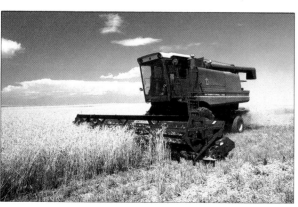

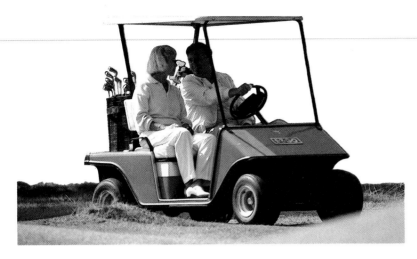

## Mechanization

Forklifts replaced longshoremen, combines and mechanical plows took a lot of the physical labor out of farm work, power saws were used for logging, and diesel engines put stokers out of work. Machines were invented to wash clothes and dishes, to clean and polish floors, and to chop and grind meat. Automobiles became the way to travel, and young people learned to regard the car (and a license to drive) as an essential social asset. Power mowers were used in the backyard, and electric-powered carts became commonplace on the golf course. All this was called progress and few people realized at first that the machine age might indirectly be a threat to health.

**Desirable or undesirable innovations?**
*Walking instead of using a cart on the golf course can help provide the physical exertion that is valuable for your health.*

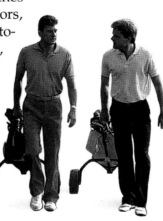

## THE PROTECTIVE EFFECTS OF EXERCISE

The first hints that an easy life might be a dangerous one came from a research study by Jerry Morris, a professor at the London School of Hygiene

**Walk or drive?**
*Walking has helped people stay healthy for generations, but today many car owners walk no more than a few hundred yards a day.*

and Tropical Medicine. He examined the health of bus workers employed on the famous red double-decker London buses and found that the drivers, who sat down all day, had more heart attacks than the conductors, who spent their working day climbing up and down stairs to collect fares.

## San Francisco longshoremen

An equally influential study was done by Ralph Paffenbarger Jr, Professor of Epidemiology at Stanford University, who studied longshoremen in San Francisco. He measured the physical energy expenditure of longshoremen who were performing different tasks on the docks. Paffenbarger showed convincingly that those whose work was consistently physically demanding had fewer cases of heart disease than those who spent their days working in supervisory or other less physically challenging positions.

Further research by Morris and Paffenbarger focused on the leisure activities of men who were employed in sedentary occupations. This study showed a clear association between regular, vigorous physical activity in the evenings and on weekends, and relative freedom from heart disease along with lower death rates.

## Lifelong habits

In yet another study, 50,000 men who were former students of Harvard University and the University of Pennsylvania were interviewed about their athletic activities, first as young men, and then regularly throughout their

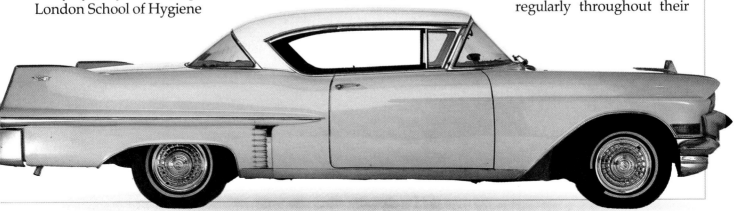

lives. A physical activity index was calculated from the energy that they spent each week in a variety of activities, including participation in light and vigorous sports. Men with low activity indexes had about 40 percent more heart attacks than those with high activity indexes.

The value of exercise became even clearer when the men's athletic activities in early life were taken into account. Half the former varsity athletes had maintained their physical interests throughout their adult lives, and these were the healthiest men in the study. A surprising finding was that those who had given up sports in their 20s had slightly higher rates of heart disease than those who had never taken up sports at all. A major conclusion of this study was that physical activity maintained throughout adult life offers considerable protection against heart disease in middle age. However, more recent studies have shown that you can benefit from regular exercise, and improve your overall fitness, no matter what age you are when you start.

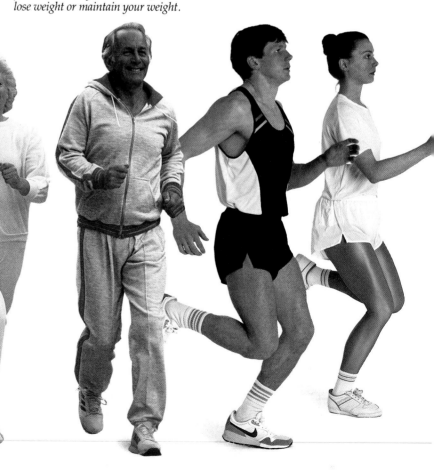

**Motivating yourself**
*There are many reasons people take up exercise. One incentive is the strong evidence that exercise helps prevent coronary heart disease; another is the desire to lose weight or maintain your weight.*

## Exercise promotes health

The findings of these and similar research studies provided a basis for recommending regular exercise as an effective form of preventive medicine. During the 1960s and 1970s, as more and more people took up jogging, walking, and aerobics, it became fashionable to participate in these activities. By the early 1990s, the need for regular exercise had become firmly established in the public consciousness. As more research is performed, doctors now believe that physical activity helps decrease the risk of chronic disease. The precise amount and type of exercise and the ways it affects health need further study.

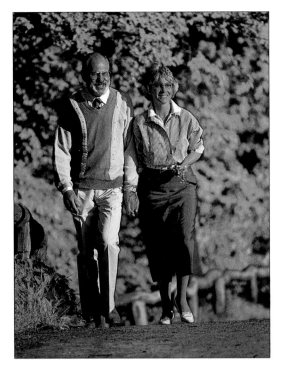

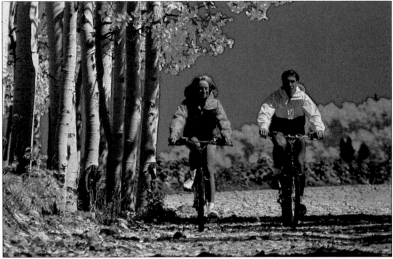

Few injuries are associated with regular brisk walking, but most runners, joggers, tennis players, and golfers have occasional injuries. However, most are not serious or long-lasting. In general, the benefits of regular exercise clearly outweigh any disadvantages.

## EXERCISE AND EVERYDAY LIFE

It was long thought that exercise had to be strenuous and make you sweaty and breathless to be effective. However, several recent research studies have shown that death rates associated with moderate levels of physical fitness are much lower than those associated with low levels of physical fitness. A good example of moderate physical activity that can make a difference in your life expectancy would be 30 to 45 minutes of brisk walking for 5 to 6 days a week.

The ideal exercise is the one that you find enjoyable. So, if you really like golf, play plenty of it, but don't use a cart. Try to make your game more physically demanding, and consider walking and carrying your clubs yourself. The ma-chines sold for home exercise can help you integrate exercise into your daily life – you can easily work up a sweat on an exercise bicycle or a rowing machine. But remember that you must be determined and stay in the habit of using the exercise equipment.

## Active alternatives

There are also many things you can do to gradually increase the level of physical activity in your everyday life. Why not walk up the stairs at the office instead of taking the elevator, or use a bicycle rather than a car for short trips? Or you could walk a few blocks rather than take the subway. All these activities will help you stay physically fit. To make sure that you are ready to walk or climb stairs, wear comfortable walking shoes that enable you to walk briskly, comfortably, and more often.

The overall message is clear – people need physical activity to maintain health. The heart, lungs, blood vessels, muscles, bones, joints, and psyche all benefit from regular exertion. Anyone whose daily routine is not physically demanding needs exercise to stay healthy.

**Avoiding passivity**
*There are many ways to avoid the easy option in your daily activities. Walking or riding a bike helps keep your heart, lungs, and muscles active and working. Also, by choosing the stairs rather than the elevator, you give yourself an excellent opportunity for valuable physical exercise.*

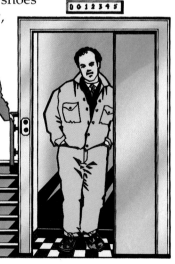

# HOW EXERCISE AFFECTS YOUR BODY

Building an exercise routine into your life may be the most positive step you can take to ensure that you will stay healthy in the years ahead. This is because certain forms of exercise bring about short- and long-term changes that improve the overall efficiency of your body and help it resist disease. When you exercise, your body must work harder than when you are relaxing. The mechanisms by which your nervous system speeds up your body are complex, but they include the release of the hormones epinephrine and norepinephrine from nerve endings and from the adrenal glands. These chemicals have a stimulating effect that causes changes to occur in many different parts of the body.

## THE BODY AT REST

### Your heart
*By pumping blood through your blood vessels, your heart ensures that all the organs and tissues are supplied with oxygen and nutrients. Normally, the heart at rest pumps about 9 pints (4 liters) of blood around the body every minute.*

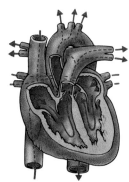

### Your lungs
*At rest, about 12 pints (6 liters) of air pass in and out of your lungs every minute. Oxygen passes into the bloodstream and is pumped to all parts of the body; waste carbon dioxide from the muscle cells returns via the blood to the lungs and is exhaled.*

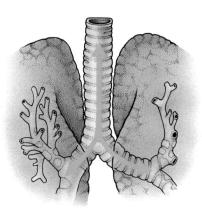

### Your digestive system
*After meals the blood supply to the digestive system is maximized as the blood vessels leading to the stomach and other parts of the digestive tract dilate (widen).*

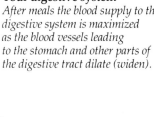

### Your muscles
*The energy requirement of your muscles is at its minimum when the muscles are at rest. Much of the blood supply is diverted elsewhere in the body to carry out functions such as digesting food.*

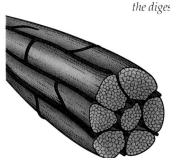

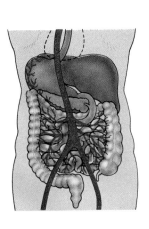

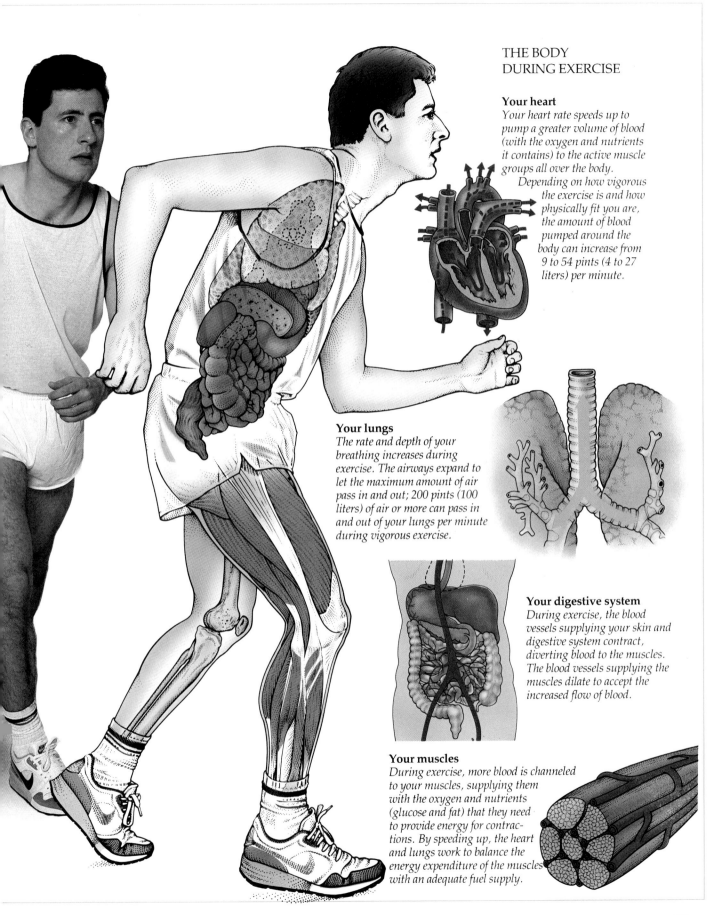

## THE BODY DURING EXERCISE

### Your heart
*Your heart rate speeds up to pump a greater volume of blood (with the oxygen and nutrients it contains) to the active muscle groups all over the body.*

*Depending on how vigorous the exercise is and how physically fit you are, the amount of blood pumped around the body can increase from 9 to 54 pints (4 to 27 liters) per minute.*

### Your lungs
*The rate and depth of your breathing increases during exercise. The airways expand to let the maximum amount of air pass in and out; 200 pints (100 liters) of air or more can pass in and out of your lungs per minute during vigorous exercise.*

### Your digestive system
*During exercise, the blood vessels supplying your skin and digestive system contract, diverting blood to the muscles. The blood vessels supplying the muscles dilate to accept the increased flow of blood.*

### Your muscles
*During exercise, more blood is channeled to your muscles, supplying them with the oxygen and nutrients (glucose and fat) that they need to provide energy for contractions. By speeding up, the heart and lungs work to balance the energy expenditure of the muscles with an adequate fuel supply.*

During an isolated session of exercise, temporary changes occur in the body. However, these changes have little or no long-term effect on the body. But when exercise is carried out on a regular basis for a prolonged time period, the body responds in several ways. Most notable are the changes that gradually take place in the muscles, including the heart muscle.

Moreover, it is important that you persevere with a regular exercise routine because the beneficial changes brought about by exercise are quickly reversed if you return to inactivity.

## YOUR HEART

Regular exercise over a prolonged period of time actually causes the heart muscle to enlarge. While the chambers inside the heart remain much the same size, the muscle fibers in the walls surrounding the chambers thicken and strengthen. The heart of a physically fit person is therefore able to pump a much larger volume of blood during a minute of exercise than the heart of a person who does not exercise regularly.

### A more powerful heart

One measure of the efficiency of the heart is stroke volume, which is the volume of blood moved by each contraction. The cardiac output is obtained by multiplying stroke volume by number of contractions per minute. The more you exert yourself, the greater the stroke volume.

A healthy heart works at rest at a rate of around 60 to 70 beats per minute, and the cardiac output may reach 9 pints (4 liters) per minute. During vigorous exercise, your heart rate (pulse) can speed up to 200 beats per minute and your cardiac output may reach 54 pints (27 liters) a minute. People in good condition tend to have a slower pulse at rest than those in poor physical condition; however, each slower heartbeat forces a greater volume of blood through the

**Exercise and the heart muscle**
*In response to the increased demands made on your heart by exercise, the fibers of your heart muscle become stronger and thicker. This more powerful action and your faster heartbeat enable the heart to pump more blood per minute. The heart functions more efficiently, both at rest and during exercise.*

**Myocardium (heart muscle)**

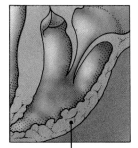

**Heart wall of a person with a sedentary life**

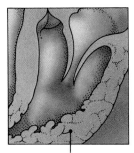

**Heart wall of a person who exercises often**

circulatory system. Some professional athletes have a heart rate as low as 40 beats per minute. However, the pulse of an out-of-condition person may be as high as 80 to 100 beats per minute.

Another sign of a healthy heart is the time it takes for the heart rate to return to its resting level after exercise. The more physically fit you are, the more quickly your heart returns to its resting level.

## YOUR LUNGS

The improvement in the overall efficiency of your heart and lungs as the result of doing regular exercise can be demonstrated in an exercise laboratory by measuring the maximum volume of oxygen ($V_{O_2}$ max) that you are capable of taking in and using in a minute during a specific strenuous exertion. A 15- to 20-week exercise program can increase your $V_{O_2}$ max by as much as 20 percent if you start exercising after a period of inactivity. However, if you stop exercising, most of this improvement in your lung capacity will disappear within 3 months.

## CHANGES THAT OCCUR IN YOUR MUSCLES

Most exercises involve frequent and rapid contractions and relaxations of muscle groups all over your body. Muscle cells require energy to contract, and this energy is gained by burning fats and glucose provided by the bloodstream. Over time, repeated exercise causes several significant changes to occur in your muscles. The changes allow a greater volume of blood into the muscle, and the muscle cells are better able to store and utilize the energy that the blood provides. The mitochondria (below) play a vital role in energy production.

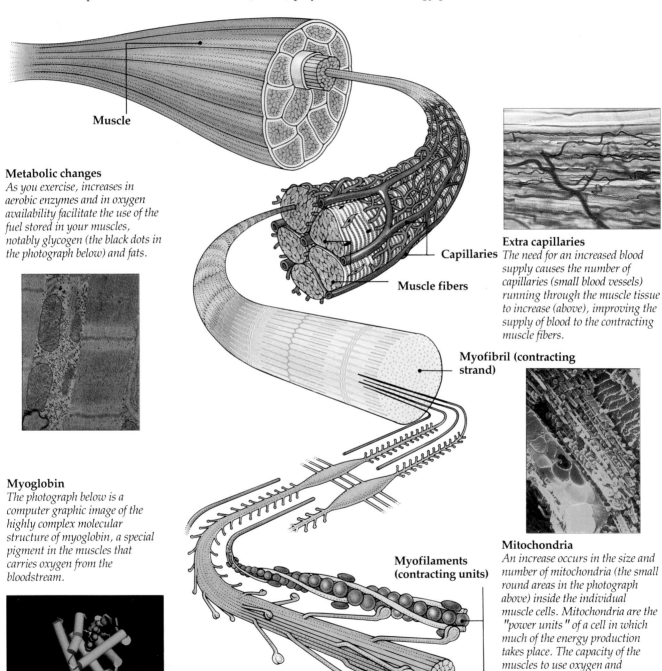

**Muscle**

**Metabolic changes**
*As you exercise, increases in aerobic enzymes and in oxygen availability facilitate the use of the fuel stored in your muscles, notably glycogen (the black dots in the photograph below) and fats.*

**Capillaries**

**Muscle fibers**

**Extra capillaries** *The need for an increased blood supply causes the number of capillaries (small blood vessels) running through the muscle tissue to increase (above), improving the supply of blood to the contracting muscle fibers.*

**Myofibril (contracting strand)**

**Myoglobin**
*The photograph below is a computer graphic image of the highly complex molecular structure of myoglobin, a special pigment in the muscles that carries oxygen from the bloodstream.*

**Myofilaments (contracting units)**

**Mitochondria**
*An increase occurs in the size and number of mitochondria (the small round areas in the photograph above) inside the individual muscle cells. Mitochondria are the "power units" of a cell in which much of the energy production takes place. The capacity of the muscles to use oxygen and produce energy is enhanced when more mitochondria are present.*

17

# THE BENEFITS OF EXERCISE

If the benefits of regular exercise were limited to the overall development of more efficient body systems, such as better breathing and stronger muscles, few people would work at it seriously or for long. In fact, many of us are motivated to exercise by the greatly improved quality of life that being in good shape can offer. Exercise can be uplifting to your mental health, and the physical changes that exercise brings can help you take more pride in your appearance.

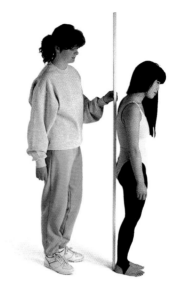

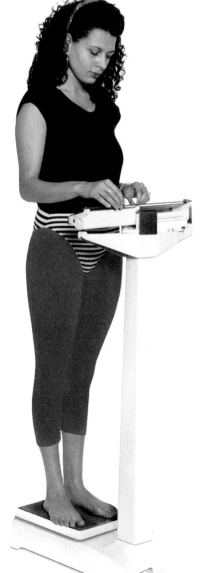

**Improved posture**
As you increase the strength and tone of your abdominal muscles and start to lose fat, you may notice an improvement in your posture (above, left and right). Stronger stomach muscles help give you better posture and may help reduce back pain.

**Weight reduction**
Exercising along with a balanced diet helps you control your weight and lose any extra pounds. Exercise increases your body's need for energy, and some of this requirement is provided by reserves of stored excess fat. Remember that you may not lose weight when you first start an exercise program. The exercise is building your muscles, and this added weight might offset the weight lost in fat. Your muscles do not necessarily get bigger (depending on the type of exercises you do), but your muscles do become more toned, which, with the loss of fat, helps you look trimmer.

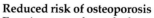

**Reduced risk of osteoporosis**
Exercise strengthens the bones by increasing their mineral content, especially their calcium content. Exercise, particularly weight-bearing exercises such as brisk walking, can also help prevent the onset of osteoporosis (progressive thinning of bone caused by calcium depletion) later in life. This is especially important for women, who become more vulnerable to osteoporosis after the menopause.

### Reduced risk of heart disease

Doing a moderate amount of exercise on a regular basis can significantly reduce your chances of having a fatal heart attack. Exercise apparently reduces the risk of coronary heart disease by helping to prevent obesity and high blood pressure and by improving blood flow through the coronary arteries. Furthermore, exercise affects the character of your blood cholesterol by reducing the level of low density lipoproteins and raising the level of high density lipoproteins. Low density lipoproteins are responsible for depositing fat into the lining of the arteries and thus play a major part in atherosclerosis, the narrowing of arteries that can lead to the formation of a blood clot and to a heart attack or stroke. High density lipoproteins, on the other hand, help prevent atherosclerosis because they act as scavengers of the fat deposited on arteries.

### Relief from anxiety and depression

You may find that regular exercise improves your sense of well-being and your self-image, making you feel brighter, more relaxed, and healthier. Exercising helps some people feel more in control of their lives. It can also bring about a natural "high" that is caused by the release of endorphins (morphinelike substances) inside your brain.

### Sound sleep and prevention of insomnia

Exercise encourages the kind of deep, refreshing sleep from which you wake relaxed and energized. Do not exercise just before bedtime; allow at least 1 hour before you go to sleep. Late afternoon may be the best time for exercise if you want to use it as a method of preventing insomnia. For best results, control your caffeine intake in the evenings, too.

### Incentive to quit smoking

Some people find that an increase in physical activity successfully motivates them to quit smoking.

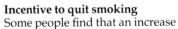

### Relief of menstrual problems

For some women, regular exercise helps reduce the severity of premenstrual symptoms and often helps ease menstrual pain.

### CANCER PREVENTION

Regular exercise has been suggested as a protection against certain cancers. In one study, cancer death rates were much lower in men and women who were physically fit. Other research studies have confirmed this link between cancer rates and levels of physical fitness.

# TYPES OF EXERCISE

Not all forms of exercise offer the same health benefits, so it is important to understand what each type of exercise can provide. Exercises may be aerobic or anaerobic. Also, there are many specialized routines designed for specific goals, such as increasing your muscle strength, rather than your overall fitness.

The term aerobic exercise is used to describe any form of prolonged activity that can be done continuously for at least 12 minutes and that uses oxygen to provide energy for the muscles. Aerobic exercises generally involve the large muscles in your trunk, upper body, and legs.

## CHOOSING A FORM OF AEROBIC EXERCISE

Many of the physical activities people do are aerobic, including brisk walking, jogging, swimming, and cycling. Regardless of the type of exercise you choose, stay within your limits, begin slowly, and gradually build up your speed and distance over several weeks.

The total amount of energy you expend is an important factor in exercise; intensity is relatively unimportant. The best exercise for you is the one that you enjoy and that you will do regularly.

### Brisk walking
One of the easiest forms of aerobic exercise is brisk walking; the number of people walking for fitness is rapidly increasing. Walking can be easily incorporated into your daily routine by walking part of the distance to your place of work and to the stores in your neighborhood. Also, encourage the children in your family to walk to school and to the park, to help them develop the habit of walking.

At first, walking only a short distance may make you feel out of breath. However, as you become conditioned, you should be able to walk farther and for longer periods. You can then start thinking about tackling a few hills, if there are any in your area. Your goal should be at least three half-hour brisk walks each week, unless you do some other form of aerobic exercise as well.

### Jogging
If you prefer to jog, build up to it gradually by walking until you can cover 2 miles without difficulty. Then alternate jogging and walking in 100-yard stretches. As you build up your endurance, you can gradually increase the distance you jog, until you are running the whole time.

To make jogging more interesting, use different routes and run at different times of the day. Try to build up to at least three or four 20-minute runs a week. Shoes that fit well and offer good arch support are important (see HOW TO CHOOSE YOUR EXERCISE SHOES on page 78).

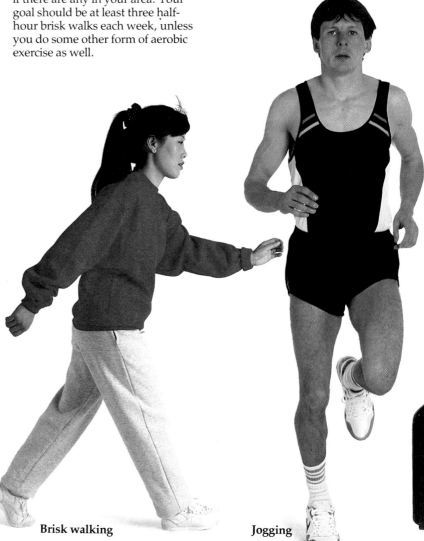

**Brisk walking**

**Jogging**

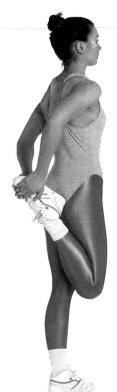

**Quadriceps**
*By holding your leg behind you and gently pulling, you can stretch the quadriceps muscle at the front of your thigh. Take care, because using an arm to help you stretch your leg can cause you to overstretch. Again, use common sense when deciding if you should try this exercise.*

**Inner parts of the thighs**
*Stand with your legs apart and move one leg away from you to the side. Then lean the upper part of your body in the opposite direction from the outstretched leg. This stretch improves flexibility in the inner thigh muscles.*

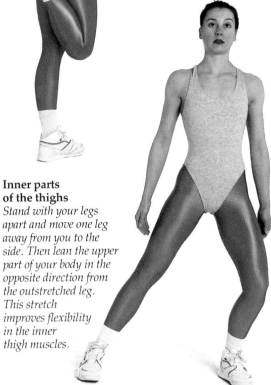

## WARNING

To avoid injury, use only slow, careful movements in your stretching exercises. Never jerk or bounce while stretching because you could injure your joint ligaments or the discs in your spine. Stretching exercises that require extra caution include
◆ leaning forward while standing or twisting
◆ high kicks
◆ twisting to one side with both feet flat on the ground
◆ deep squats
◆ vigorous neck stretching
◆ kneeling thigh stretch
◆ sitting hurdle stretch, with knee bent under you
◆ touching your toes (use a smooth motion; never bounce your body or jerk suddenly).

## YOGA

Many people have adopted yoga as an exercise program. Yoga teaches relaxation and breathing control through a series of positions, known as postures, that exercise virtually every part of the body. It is best to begin a yoga program very carefully in a class supervised by a qualified teacher; some positions may lead to overstretching and injury if done incorrectly. In some communities, special yoga classes are taught for the elderly, and some yoga positions are modified, or not done at all, to minimize the risk of injury. Middle-aged people should also be cautious about starting yoga and experimenting with positions.

**The art of yoga**
*Yoga has many benefits. It produces an excellent degree of suppleness, improves endurance, and (to a lesser degree) improves strength. Done correctly, yoga clears the mind and produces a feeling of relaxation. It is noncompetitive and safe for all ages when caution is observed with some of the more demanding positions.*

**Abdomen**
*This stretch from a kneeling position strengthens the muscles that cover the front of the abdomen. In step 3, stretch to the point where you feel a pull in the muscle, and hold this stretch for a count of 10. In time you will be able to hold yourself in the position for up to 30 seconds.*

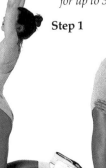 **Step 1**
 **Step 2**
 **Step 3**

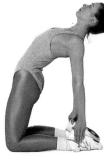

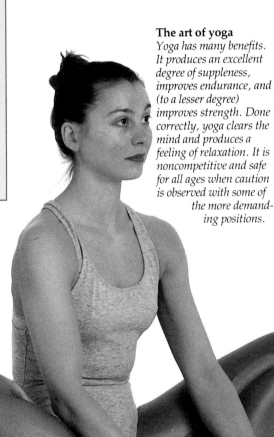

# STRENGTH EXERCISES

Your body contains a few hundred different muscles, and you can exercise to strengthen each group. Strength exercises may be dynamic, in which the muscles change in length, or isometric, in which the muscle contracts without shortening. No visible movement accompanies isometrics. For example, pushing your palms against each other is isometric exercise for the muscles in your arms. Dynamic exercise is further subdivided into isotonic exercises, where the length of the muscle changes but the tension remains more or less constant, and isokinetic exercises, which use special equipment to maintain mechanical tension against the muscles.

## Dynamic muscle exercises

The most effective and safe form of dynamic exercise involves repeated movement against a force, usually in the form of a weight, springs, hydraulic valves, or elastic tubing. To increase the strength and tone of your muscles, you need not move heavy weights. Start with weights you find relatively easy to move and build up gradually. Hold weights at

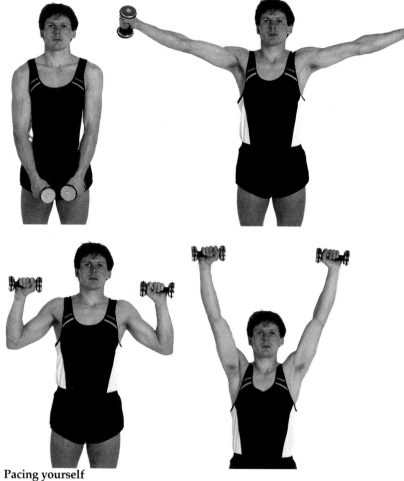

**Pacing yourself**
*The weights you use while exercising should be small enough for you to complete at least eight repetitions. Increase the number of repetitions before you add weight, aiming to build up to 12 repetitions over a 60-second period. If you can do three*

*sets of 15 repetitions on one muscle group without any difficulty, you are ready to increase the load. Remember that it is more important to perform the movement correctly than it is to do as many repetitions as you can in as short a time as possible.*

**Increasing muscle bulk**
*All muscles increase in size if exercised regularly, although some exercises have a more pronounced effect than others. Although the number of muscle fibers apparently remains the same, an increase occurs in the number of myofibrils (contracting strands) inside the fibers. The fibers thus become thicker. Through exercise, expansion also occurs in the tendons and tissue that envelops the muscle.*

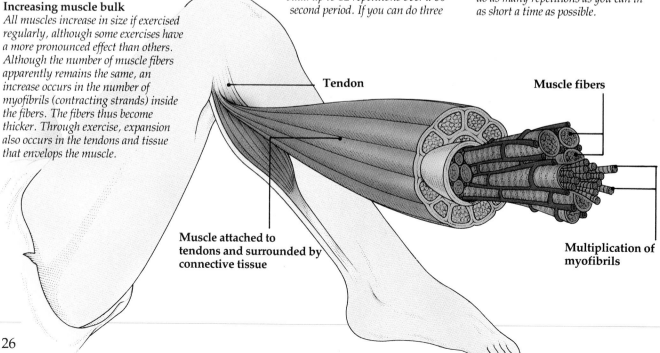

**Tendon**

**Muscle fibers**

**Muscle attached to tendons and surrounded by connective tissue**

**Multiplication of myofibrils**

the farthest point from the center of the movement for a count of two and breathe out at the same time.

Ideally, dynamic exercises should be started under supervision. Your instructor can recommend a range of exercises, each one working a specific group of muscles, and can ensure that you are performing the movements correctly to minimize your risk of injury.

## Muscle bulk

Repeated dynamic exercises using small weights improve muscle strength and tone without dramatically increasing the size of your muscles. The lack of the male hormone testosterone prevents such a muscle buildup for women using small loads.

**Heavy weights**
*For many people, lifting heavy weights repeatedly is not a useful exercise. When you do a series of lifts, the exercise is anaerobic, increasing the lactic acid in your muscles. Also, a weight-lifting series does not increase the efficiency of your heart and lungs. The weight lifter also has a high risk of injury.*

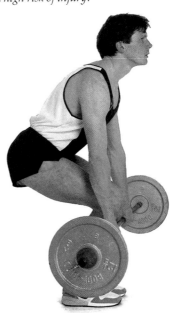

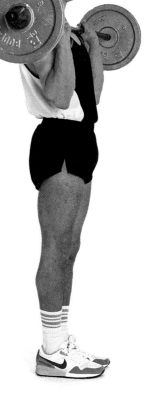

**Step 1**

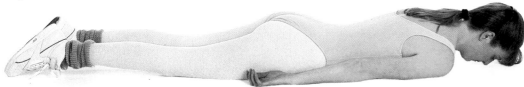

**Step 2**

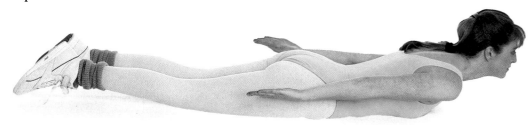

**Step 3**

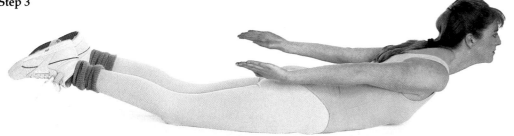

**Isometric exercises**
*Do isometric muscle-strengthening exercises, in which the muscle contracts without changing its length, by using one part of your body to resist the movement of another part. A form of resistance is not always necessary. In step 3 of the routine shown at left, several muscle groups are exercised isometrically as you hold your body in position with the legs raised for a period of time. Note that isometric exercise tends to increase blood pressure.*

# CHOOSING YOUR EXERCISE

If you have a job that involves sitting behind a desk, a car to take you wherever you want to go, and a TV, video-cassette recorder, or stereo to enjoy when you get home, exercise may not be an everyday part of your life. Most people are aware of the importance of exercising regularly but many of us have a problem finding the time or the motivation to get started and deciding which form of exercise to try.

## EXERCISING AT HOME

Exercising at home is a convenient way of making sure that you work out regularly without compromising your other commitments. Many people also prefer to exercise in the privacy of their home until they feel they are more in shape and therefore ready to join others in a social setting while exercising.

### Finding out what suits you

You can try some types of exercise at home without using any special equipment. For other types of exercise you may simply adapt ordinary furniture or parts of the building structure. For example, you can use chairs, walls, and door frames to provide support.

You may decide that purchasing a piece of equipment will offer more chances to exercise. The advantage of having your own machine at home is convenience. Devices such as exercise bicycles, treadmills, and rowing, skiing, and stair-climbing machines effectively simulate the physical experience of some popular outdoor activities. Regular use of exercise equipment will produce beneficial effects on your health. However, before you buy an expensive piece of equipment, try out the available models.

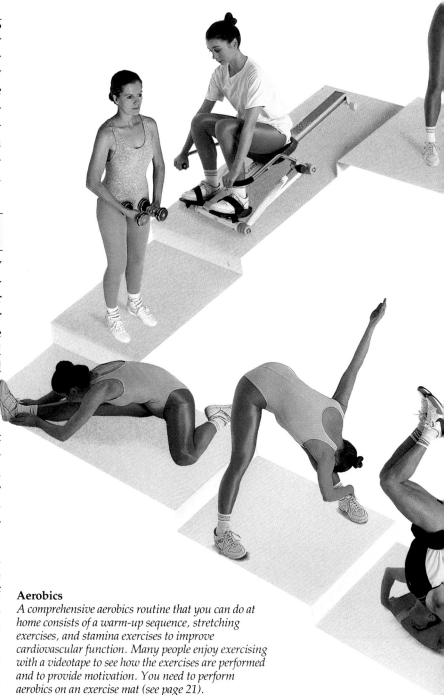

**Convenience and privacy**
*The use of exercise machines at home is very popular. The machines range from fairly simple devices to more sophisticated ones that use a computer to monitor your progress. Many people feel self-conscious about exercising in front of strangers at a health club and enjoy the privacy at home.*

**Aerobics**
*A comprehensive aerobics routine that you can do at home consists of a warm-up sequence, stretching exercises, and stamina exercises to improve cardiovascular function. Many people enjoy exercising with a videotape to see how the exercises are performed and to provide motivation. You need to perform aerobics on an exercise mat (see page 21).*

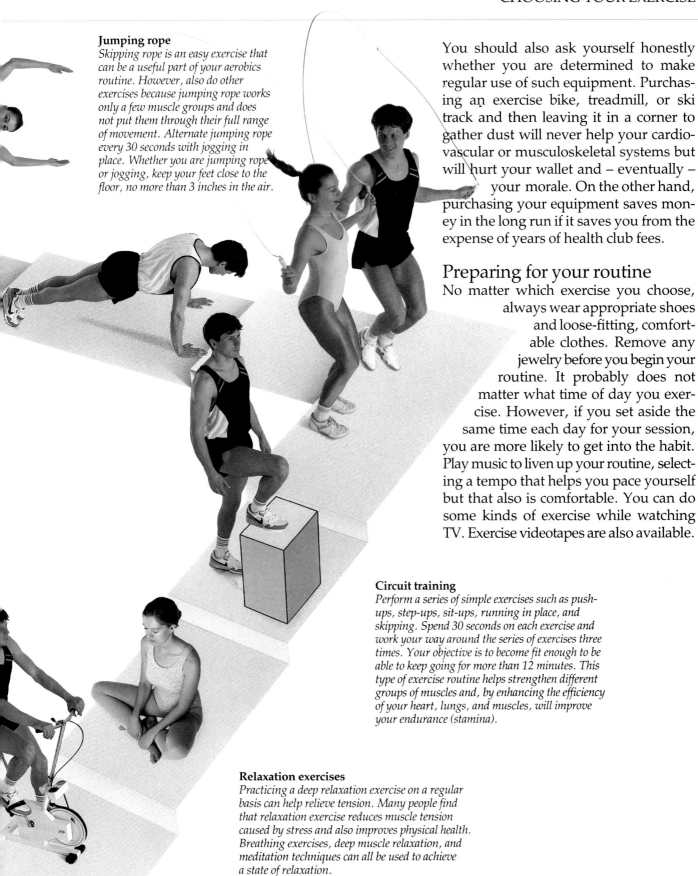

### Jumping rope

*Skipping rope is an easy exercise that can be a useful part of your aerobics routine. However, also do other exercises because jumping rope works only a few muscle groups and does not put them through their full range of movement. Alternate jumping rope every 30 seconds with jogging in place. Whether you are jumping rope or jogging, keep your feet close to the floor, no more than 3 inches in the air.*

You should also ask yourself honestly whether you are determined to make regular use of such equipment. Purchasing an exercise bike, treadmill, or ski track and then leaving it in a corner to gather dust will never help your cardiovascular or musculoskeletal systems but will hurt your wallet and – eventually – your morale. On the other hand, purchasing your equipment saves money in the long run if it saves you from the expense of years of health club fees.

## Preparing for your routine

No matter which exercise you choose, always wear appropriate shoes and loose-fitting, comfortable clothes. Remove any jewelry before you begin your routine. It probably does not matter what time of day you exercise. However, if you set aside the same time each day for your session, you are more likely to get into the habit. Play music to liven up your routine, selecting a tempo that helps you pace yourself but that also is comfortable. You can do some kinds of exercise while watching TV. Exercise videotapes are also available.

### Circuit training

*Perform a series of simple exercises such as push-ups, step-ups, sit-ups, running in place, and skipping. Spend 30 seconds on each exercise and work your way around the series of exercises three times. Your objective is to become fit enough to be able to keep going for more than 12 minutes. This type of exercise routine helps strengthen different groups of muscles and, by enhancing the efficiency of your heart, lungs, and muscles, will improve your endurance (stamina).*

### Relaxation exercises

*Practicing a deep relaxation exercise on a regular basis can help relieve tension. Many people find that relaxation exercise reduces muscle tension caused by stress and also improves physical health. Breathing exercises, deep muscle relaxation, and meditation techniques can all be used to achieve a state of relaxation.*

## EXERCISING WITH OTHER PEOPLE

Many people find that the main problem with exercise is not what to do or how to do it, but how to keep doing it regularly. Taking up an activity or sport that involves other people – perhaps your friends or colleagues at work – may help you continue your exercising, despite any lapses in willpower that you might experience. Friends may not let you quit so easily, and you will encourage each other to meet and get involved on a regular basis if you join a volleyball team or set a regular date each week for golfing. Alternatively, you can join a health club and exercise or play a sport with other members of the club.

Many adults take evening or weekend exercise classes at schools or community centers. Encourage the children and the adolescents in your family to join you in an exercise class and to participate in team sports whenever possible.

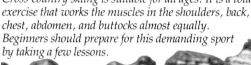

**Cross-country skiing – a growing sport**
*Cross-country skiing is suitable for all ages. It is a total exercise that works the muscles in the shoulders, back, chest, abdomen, and buttocks almost equally. Beginners should prepare for this demanding sport by taking a few lessons.*

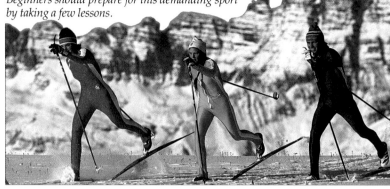

**Team sports**
*Playing competitive team sports such as basketball keeps you involved in fitness activities on a regular basis. Friendly golf games or tennis matches against players of similar ability are more satisfying for some people than a solitary regimen at a health club. Your age, your competitive spirit, and your level of fitness should influence your choice.*

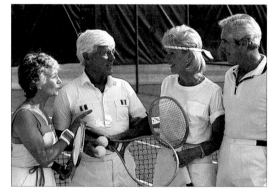

### What exercises are people choosing?

Group exercises are a fun and sociable way to get and stay in shape for many people. Your choice of activity will depend in part on your age, level of fitness, and exercise goals. A game of racquetball or a challenging round of golf, without a cart, can be a sociable form of exercise for adults, while roller-skating or ice-skating may be preferred by teenagers or young adults in your family.

In recent years, the number of people participating in socially oriented exercise, such as tennis, cross-country skiing, and cycling, has greatly increased. This trend may reflect the fact that many people work long hours and are looking for ways to combine fitness with social activity. Many exercises can be enjoyed by most family members. Participating in exercises and sports as a family unit or with friends can be healthy, convenient, and satisfying.

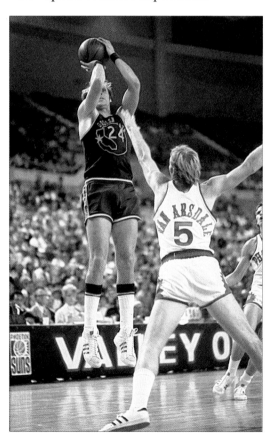

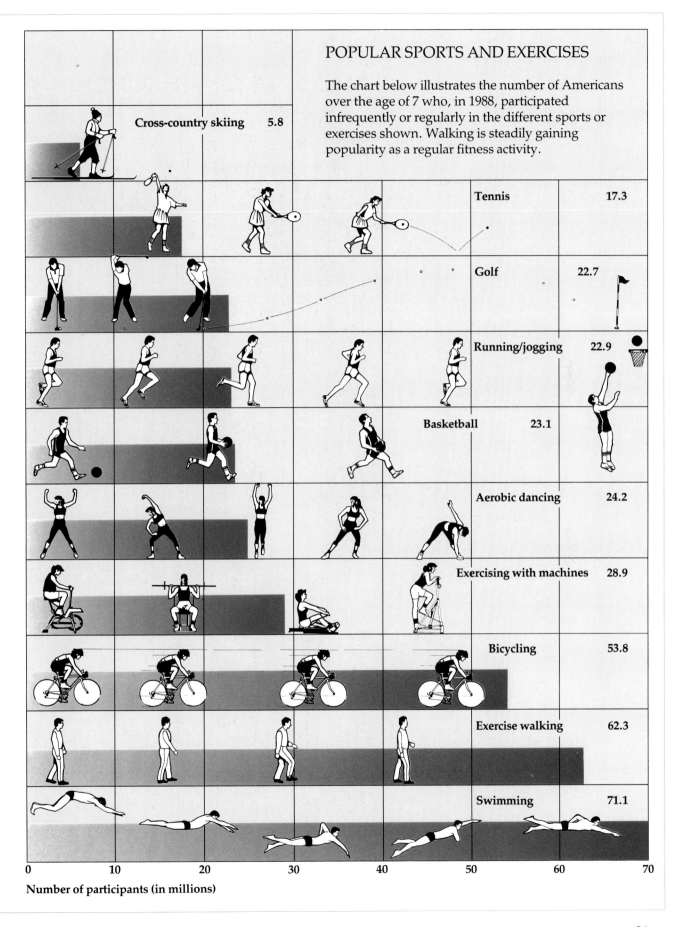

## POPULAR SPORTS AND EXERCISES

The chart below illustrates the number of Americans over the age of 7 who, in 1988, participated infrequently or regularly in the different sports or exercises shown. Walking is steadily gaining popularity as a regular fitness activity.

| Sport/Exercise | Participants (millions) |
|---|---|
| Cross-country skiing | 5.8 |
| Tennis | 17.3 |
| Golf | 22.7 |
| Running/jogging | 22.9 |
| Basketball | 23.1 |
| Aerobic dancing | 24.2 |
| Exercising with machines | 28.9 |
| Bicycling | 53.8 |
| Exercise walking | 62.3 |
| Swimming | 71.1 |

**Number of participants (in millions)**

0    10    20    30    40    50    60    70

## EXERCISING AT A HEALTH CLUB

Although people go to a health club or gym for many types of exercise, in recent years many have joined health clubs specifically to exercise with the mechanical weight-lifting apparatus. These machines strengthen specific groups of muscles and are safer than free weights because they eliminate the risk of dropping a weight on yourself or falling with a weight in your arms.

### Supervision and safety

Ideally, a staff trainer at the health club should supervise your first session or two so that you can learn a sequence of exercises that works each muscle group of your body in turn. A supervisor should also instruct you on the proper execution of each exercise to make sure you are using the equipment safely.

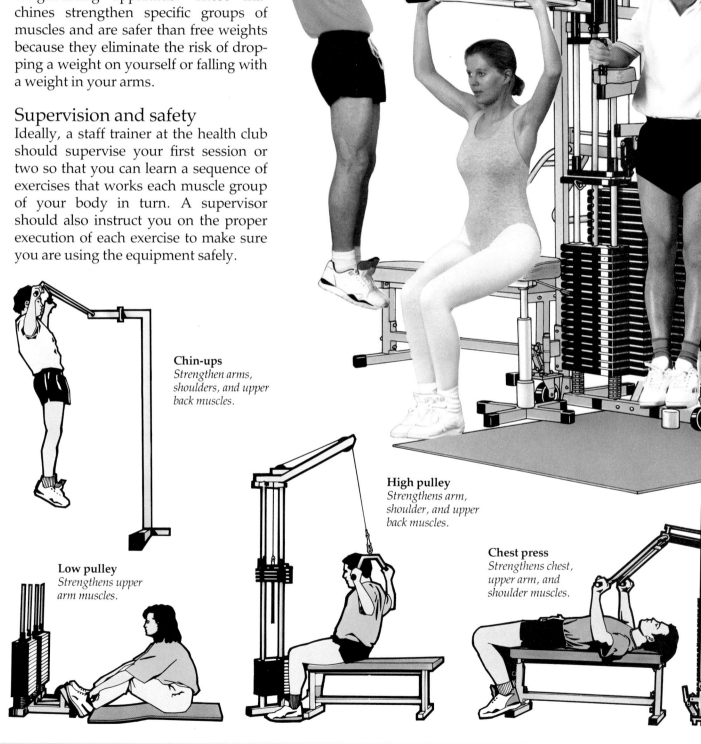

**Hip flexor**

**Chin-ups**

**Shoulder press**

**Chin-ups**
*Strengthen arms, shoulders, and upper back muscles.*

**High pulley**
*Strengthens arm, shoulder, and upper back muscles.*

**Low pulley**
*Strengthens upper arm muscles.*

**Chest press**
*Strengthens chest, upper arm, and shoulder muscles.*

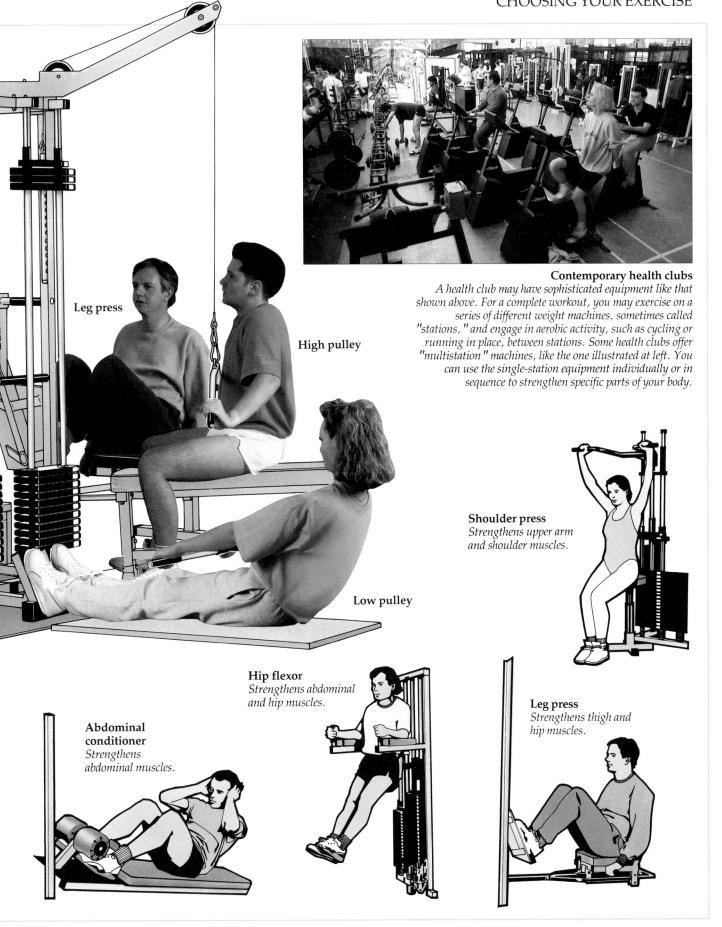

**Leg press**

**High pulley**

**Contemporary health clubs**
*A health club may have sophisticated equipment like that shown above. For a complete workout, you may exercise on a series of different weight machines, sometimes called "stations," and engage in aerobic activity, such as cycling or running in place, between stations. Some health clubs offer "multistation" machines, like the one illustrated at left. You can use the single-station equipment individually or in sequence to strengthen specific parts of your body.*

**Low pulley**

**Shoulder press**
*Strengthens upper arm and shoulder muscles.*

**Hip flexor**
*Strengthens abdominal and hip muscles.*

**Abdominal conditioner**
*Strengthens abdominal muscles.*

**Leg press**
*Strengthens thigh and hip muscles.*

33

# EXERCISE AND DIET

Some people believe that, if you exercise or play a sport, you require special food supplements to satisfy your body's increased needs for nutrients and energy. It is true that the more active you are the higher the calorie intake you will need. However, a balanced diet with a moderate intake of protein (including dairy products), plenty of whole grains (bread or cereal), fresh fruit, and vegetables should satisfy most needs. Such a diet is adequate for most people who exercise; additional vitamin or food supplements are not required to stay healthy.

## ENERGY SOURCES

When you exercise, your muscle cells get the energy to contract primarily from the breakdown of glucose and fat. Glucose is converted from glycogen, a starchy substance derived from dietary carbohydrate that is stored in the muscles and liver (see HOW DO MUSCLES GAIN THEIR ENERGY? on page 22).

When you have started to utilize your stores of glycogen, and oxygen is available in sufficient quantity, energy is also supplied by the breakdown of fat, which is stored in the muscles and in deposits under the skin. With sustained exercise, the body continues to use its stores of glycogen and fat. Therefore, if you want to lose weight, the total energy you expend during physical activity must exceed the amount of fuel (calories in food and drink) that you take in.

### Carbohydrate

The carbohydrates found in foods fall into three groups – sugar, starch, and a group consisting of cellulose and related materials. Your body breaks down sugar and starch to provide energy. Humans cannot digest cellulose but it is an important dietary fiber that helps keep your digestive system working efficiently.

## EXERCISE, FAT, AND MUSCLE

Although a single brief exercise session produces no change in muscle tissue, long-term regular exercise such as weight lifting or cycling will increase your muscle protein and thus cause an increase in your muscle size. At the same time, your stores of body fat are reduced as they are used up for energy.

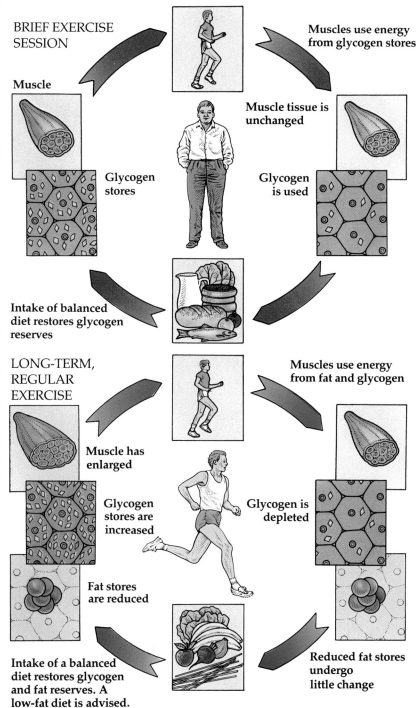

BRIEF EXERCISE SESSION

Muscle

Glycogen stores

Muscles use energy from glycogen stores

Muscle tissue is unchanged

Glycogen is used

Intake of balanced diet restores glycogen reserves

LONG-TERM, REGULAR EXERCISE

Muscle has enlarged

Glycogen stores are increased

Fat stores are reduced

Intake of a balanced diet restores glycogen and fat reserves. A low-fat diet is advised.

Muscles use energy from fat and glycogen

Glycogen is depleted

Reduced fat stores undergo little change

Sugar, which is found in foods such as fruit, milk, and sugar cane, is known as a simple carbohydrate. Starch and cellulose, which are more complex chemicals than sugar, are found in foods such as potatoes, beans, cereals, and grains.

Exercising when you feel hungry can lead to hunger pains. The best time to eat is about 3 hours before you exercise. If you eat less than an hour before, food remaining in your stomach may cause you to feel nauseous.

Exercise diverts blood flow from your digestive tract to your muscles, slowing down the rate of absorption of nutrients from the intestine into the bloodstream. Carbohydrates are the best type of food to eat before exercise for an immediate supply of energy; fat and protein are digested and absorbed more slowly.

## PROTEIN

In well-nourished people, protein is not used to any great degree by the body as an energy source during exercise. Protein provides the amino acids that are needed to build, maintain, and repair your muscle tissues. Many people in the US and other developed countries eat at least twice the recommended allowance of protein each day, yet the myth persists that protein supplementation is indispensable when they begin exercising.

## The effects of too much protein

Unless your diet is unbalanced, you are probably taking in all the protein you require for exercise. If you do muscle-building exercises, you may need to eat additional protein, which will be used by your body to form added muscle tissue. Young people who are still growing may need more protein for the added demands of sports. Under normal circumstances, however, your body can use only a limited amount of protein at a time; any surplus is broken down and the by-products are excreted in the urine.

Eating too much protein on a regular basis may cause problems for people with liver and kidney disorders by placing an unnecessary strain on these organs. However, for most people, the main argument against adopting a high-protein diet is that many meats rich in

### HOW MUCH PROTEIN IS TOO MUCH?

Your daily protein intake will be adequate if you eat from 5 to 7 ounces of cooked lean meat, poultry, fish, or an equivalent amount derived from other protein sources. For example, one egg, one half cup of cooked dry beans, or 2 tablespoons of peanut butter have the same protein content as 1 ounce of meat. Getting your protein from several different sources will help you obtain a balanced supply of amino acids and other nutrients.

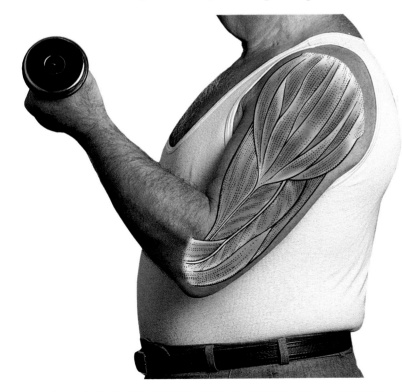

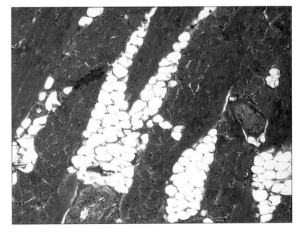

**Fat metabolism**
*The white globules lying between streaks of red muscle tissue (above) are stores of body fat. During exercise your muscle cells metabolize fat to produce energy. The metabolism of fat for energy can occur only when the necessary amount of oxygen is available in the body. To burn fat through weight lifting (left), you need to do the exercise regularly so that it becomes aerobic (uses oxygen).*

protein are also high in saturated fats. An excessive intake of these fats raises your cholesterol level and places you at an increased risk of atherosclerosis, or hardening of the arteries, which may eventually cause thrombosis (blockage) of your arteries, coronary heart disease, or stroke. Also, if you develop a habit of eating large portions of meat – particularly high-fat meats – you may be consuming more calories than you need.

## NUTRITIONAL FADS

Many nutritional products on the market are purported to provide health benefits, but such claims are unproven. There is no proof that sports drinks and high-

dose supplements of vitamins, minerals, and protein can enhance your fitness. Some nutritional supplements are even potentially harmful. Eating a varied and balanced diet is the best way to ensure that your nutritional needs are met.

## LIQUIDS

An adequate intake of liquids is essential both before and after exercise. The ideal way to drink liquids is in small amounts and at short intervals. Water is usually the best choice. You should avoid tea, coffee, and cola because they contain caffeine, which is a diuretic drug that increases your risk of dehydration by diverting body fluids into your urine. Alcohol is a poor choice, too (see A–Z OF DRUGS IN SPORTS on page 136).

PREVENTING DEHYDRATION

At least 30 minutes before exercising, drink one or two glasses of water to ensure that your tissues are adequately supplied with fluid. This is particularly important in very hot weather.

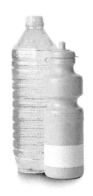

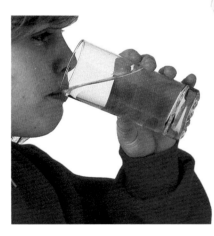

After strenuous exercise, drink water to replace fluid lost in perspiration. If you sweat a lot in this session, drink more water 30 to 45 minutes later.

**Be prepared**
*If you are exercising away from home, make sure you have access to liquids or take your own supply.*

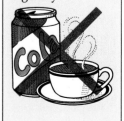

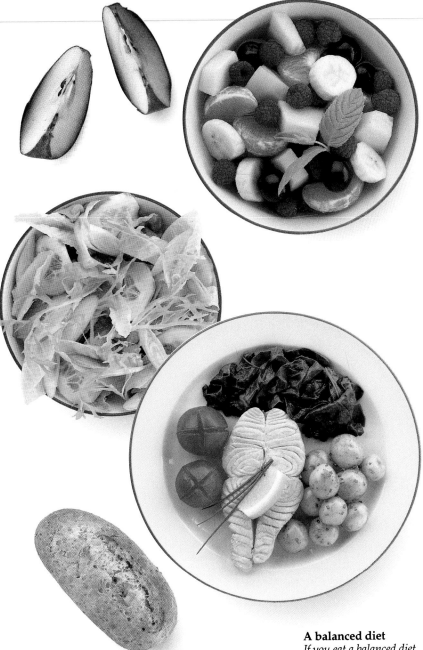

**A balanced diet**
*If you eat a balanced diet of naturally occurring foods, you don't need vitamin and mineral supplements, protein drinks, or other so-called nutritional aids. Broiled fish (above) and poultry are low in fat and are therefore popular choices among health-conscious people. A whole-grain roll adds fiber to the meal, and a fresh fruit salad is a good low-calorie dessert.*

Perspiring heavily causes you to lose fluid from your body. To counteract this loss, you should have one or two glasses of something to drink about 30 minutes before strenuous exercise. Also remember to have a drink between 30 and 45 minutes after exercising in addition to any liquid you decide to drink during or right after you finish the exercise. Feeling thirsty is not a reliable guide to the amount of fluid you have lost during a workout, so make a habit of drinking liquids while exercising, even when you are not prompted to do so by thirst.

## ASK YOUR DOCTOR
## EXERCISE AND DIET

**Q** Because I am in the service, I exercise very hard all year round. Don't I need to take vitamin and mineral supplements regularly to help my performance?

**A** No. Supplements do not improve the efficiency of your heart or muscles. In fact, excesses of vitamins A, D, E, and K accumulate in the body and can reach toxic levels that could harm your body. Eating a balanced diet that includes protein, fresh fruits and vegetables, whole grains, and dairy products is the best way to get the vitamins and minerals you need.

**Q** My daughter, who is an enthusiastic swimmer, takes iron supplements prescribed by her doctor. Why does she need them?

**A** An iron deficiency may develop in some women who are physically active, especially if they also have heavy menstrual periods. This deficiency may be confirmed by a blood test and then treated by an increased intake of iron-enriched breads and cereals, meat, fish, and poultry. Iron tablets or capsules may also be prescribed if anemia has already developed and a change in diet does not produce improvement.

**Q** Should I take amino acid supplements to stimulate muscle growth and development?

**A** No, doctors do not recommend this. Two amino acids, arginine and ornithine, increase the release of growth hormone, which increases muscle size. However, you would need to take dangerously high amounts of these amino acids to increase growth hormone production.

# CHAPTER TWO

# EXERCISE IS FOR EVERYONE

INTRODUCTION

EXERCISE AND THE
HEALTHY FAMILY

EXERCISE AND BEING
OVERWEIGHT

EXERCISE AND
SICKNESS

EXERCISE SHOULD BE an important element in your life, whether you are young or old, male or female, in good health or poor health. The physical and psychological benefits of exercise have been known for a long time, yet these benefits have been neglected and undervalued by many people. Doctors now know much more about the ways in which exercise protects us from disease, and exercise is increasingly regarded as a significant factor in healthy living. Many people have developed a negative image of exercise from the way it was presented to them as children and have maintained a strong dislike for any type of physical activity. To prevent this attitude from the start, it is particularly important for children to learn to equate being physically active with having fun. When exercise becomes a pleasant habit early in life, the active child is more likely to grow into an active adult.

In this chapter, we look at how exercise benefits every member of the family, regardless of age. Children need exercise to develop a strong heart and lungs, to strengthen their muscles, to develop strong, healthy bones, and to enhance their coordination, balance, speed, and flexibility. Pregnant women who exer-

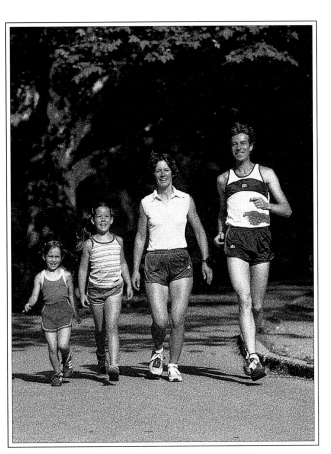

cise regularly are likely to have fewer problems during pregnancy and an easier labor. And regular exercise is also important for older people because it can slow down the natural degeneration of the muscles, tendons, ligaments, bones, and joints, as well as help maintain mobility, strength, balance, and coordination, thus reducing the risk of a fall. We also examine the advantages of physical exercise for an overweight person. Many people do not realize that regular low-intensity exercise can – in connection with a reduced-calorie balanced diet – help them lose weight. Finally, we review exercise and sickness. Many diseases and conditions, including back pain, arthritis, high blood pressure, diabetes, and some heart conditions, can be improved by appropriate exercise. You may have a condition (such as asthma or Parkinson's disease) that is not actually improved by exercise, but still it is important for you to exercise to maintain overall physical fitness and mobility. A word of caution – conditions such as anemia, some heart problems, and epilepsy require special precautions when you exercise. This chapter provides exercise guidelines for people who have these diseases and disorders.

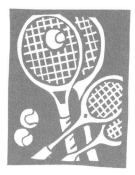

# EXERCISE AND THE HEALTHY FAMILY

WELL-ESTABLISHED exercise habits play an important part in keeping every member of the family healthy. Children need exercise to develop strong hearts and lungs. Pregnant women who exercise regularly usually have easier pregnancies and labor. And older members of the family benefit greatly from keeping their bodies active, in terms of heightened physical fitness, greater flexibility and mobility, and maintaining a positive state of mind.

Physical fitness should be an essential part of everyone's life, at any age. However, at every stage of your life, exercise should be selected according to your particular state of health.

## EXERCISE AND CHILDREN

Too many children and adolescents in the US are out of shape. Although young children always seem to be on the go, many eventually fall into the habit of slumping in front of a television set as soon as they get home from school. Recent surveys have shown that most chil-

dren watch too much television. More than 20 percent of American children suffer from obesity and poor eating habits. A recent report, entitled The National Children and Youth Fitness Study, found that only about one third of children aged 10 to 17 had daily physical education classes. Parents must take responsibility for making sure their children get enough exercise.

### The benefits of exercise

With coronary heart disease causing more deaths than any other disorder, there is increasing concern that one

**"Couch potato" children**
*Too many children and adolescents spend too much time sitting passively in front of a television set and snacking. Their mental and physical health would benefit from more exercise.*

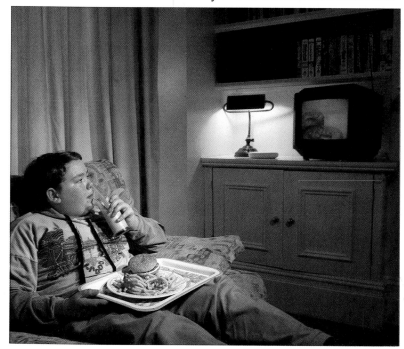

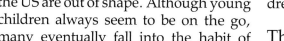

THE YOUNG ATHLETE'S
BILL OF RIGHTS

♦ The right to have the opportunity to participate in sports, regardless of the child's level of ability.
♦ The right to participate at a level commensurate with the child's level of development.
♦ The right to have qualified adult leadership.
♦ The right to participate in a safe and healthy environment.
♦ The right of each child to share leadership and decision-making.
♦ The right to play as a child and not as an adult.
♦ The right to proper preparation for participation in sports.
♦ The right to equal opportunity to strive for success.
♦ The right to be treated with dignity by all involved.
♦ The right to have fun through sports.

cause of this problem lies in lack of physical activity in childhood. A lack of exercise increases your chances of being overweight, of having abnormal blood lipid levels of cholesterol and other fats, and of suffering from high blood pressure – all risk factors for coronary heart disease that can begin to have an impact as early as the adolescent years.

Apart from promoting fitness of the heart and lungs, regular exercise also strengthens the muscles, thus helping joint stability and improving posture. In addition, exercise is considered important for the growth and development of a strong, healthy skeleton.

Along with the physical benefits, sports also help children learn to experience and manage success and failure. Participating in sports teaches them how to cooperate with their peers.

It's important that children equate being active with having fun, so try to find an activity, such as dancing or roller-skating, that your child enjoys. Most schools or local park districts sponsor after-school activities, such as soccer or tennis, for boys and girls of all ages.

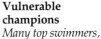

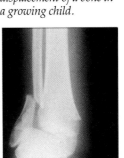

**Vulnerable champions**
*Many top swimmers, gymnasts, and tennis players are still in their teens. Their skeletons are not yet fully developed and, as a result, they are vulnerable to more serious injuries than older competitors. An accident that might sprain a ligament in an adult, for example, could instead cause a fracture or displacement of a bone in a growing child.*

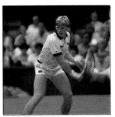

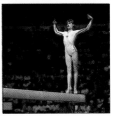

**Broken ankle**
*A broken ankle is usually caused by a hard fall at an awkward angle. Fatigue from overexercising may increase your risk of such injuries.*

**MENSTRUAL CYCLE**

Girls who train vigorously may stop having menstrual periods or delay starting them. Once a girl who already has started menstruating reduces her training schedule, her menstrual cycle usually returns to normal.

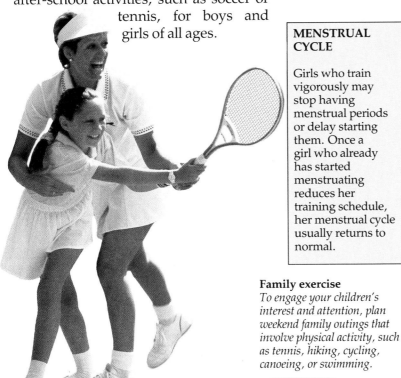

**Family exercise**
*To engage your children's interest and attention, plan weekend family outings that involve physical activity, such as tennis, hiking, cycling, canoeing, or swimming.*

## EXERCISING TOO HARD

In contrast to most children, who need prodding to do any kind of exercise, there is a small dedicated minority who spend several hours each day exercising intensely. This may be because of their own desire to excel or because overenthusiastic parents or coaches push them too hard. Loss of appetite, difficulty sleeping, and a constant feeling of exhaustion may be signs of overtraining. Children or adolescents who overtrain or overexercise may be injured or complain of stress. It is important to give children the freedom to slow down or change sports when they want to.

Some teenage athletes have been advised to take anabolic steroids to build up their muscles and improve performance generally. Steroids are extremely dangerous. They can permanently stunt growth in the developing musculoskeletal system and damage the testicles. Ask your family doctor about *any* medication recommended for your child.

# CASE HISTORY
# AN OUT-OF-CONDITION TEENAGER

**A**NGELA HAS BECOME VERY OVERWEIGHT, **largely because she prefers to spend her leisure time in front of the television rather than do any form of exercise. She is a cause of concern to her parents, especially her mother, who calls her a "couch potato." Angela's parents know that atherosclerosis, which narrows the arteries and makes them prone to obstruction, may begin soon after childhood.**

### PERSONAL DETAILS
**Name** Angela Wolff
**Age** 13
**Occupation** Student
**Family** Angela is an only child. Her parents are both in good health.

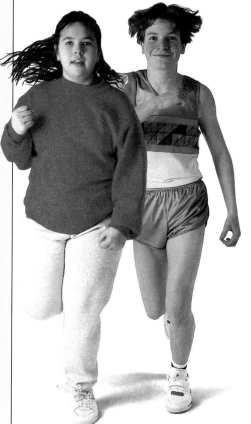

**Companionship**
*Adolescents may be motivated to exercise by the chance to be with friends their own age.*

### MEDICAL BACKGROUND
Angela is well and has had only the usual childhood diseases.

### THE PROBLEM
Even as a young child, Angela always was a plump girl, but her parents were not too worried about what they thought of as "baby fat." However, rather than becoming thinner as she got older, Angela put on more weight, which started to distress her and her parents.

Angela's parents are worried because they know that children as young as Angela often have fatty streaks in their arteries, and that these streaks can become the sites of future atherosclerosis. While they are aware that a high-fat diet is the main factor in the development of atherosclerosis, Angela's parents also know that people who exercise regularly have a better chance of avoiding this dangerous and life-shortening condition than those who are sedentary.

Although Angela's parents are healthy and conscientious about watching their weight, Angela's grandfather on her father's side of the family died of a heart attack before age 50. That early death made Angela's parents sensitive to the risk factors for heart disease.

Angela cannot be persuaded to accompany her parents on walks in the forest preserve. She considers jogging too strenuous and swimming a waste of time. Although the family eats a well-balanced diet at home, Angela spends some of her allowance on french fries on her way home from school.

### THE SOLUTION
One day, to her parents' astonishment, Angela announces that she is going roller-skating. Diplomatically, they refrain from asking her any questions, and soon afterward they are pleased to comply with her wish for a new pair of skates. A request for workout clothes soon follows. Her parents also buy her a pair of good running shoes to wear when she jogs after school.

### THE EXPLANATION
Delighted, Angela's mother finds the opportunity to talk to her about her new interests. Angela has become involved in environmental activities after school. She wants to look good and feel better around the new friends she made during a recycling project for the Earth Day committee. For a young person in her teenage years, the need for approval from her peers is a greater motivation to exercise than the seemingly distant threat of coronary heart disease.

## EXERCISE DURING PREGNANCY

Women who stay physically fit by exercising regularly tend to have easier pregnancies and labor. Women who normally do manual labor such as farm work tend to have fewer problems with childbirth, perhaps because they perform strenuous physical work and remain in good physical condition throughout pregnancy.

### Preparation

If you are planning to become pregnant, try to get in shape in advance. Pregnant women who have been inactive for several months should start with some gentle exercise, such as walking, and go slowly at first. Try to do at least a modest amount of exercise each day, rather than a lot one day and then nothing for a week. Gradually increase the distance you walk or swim, and work up to about 20 minutes at a time.

Because pregnancy temporarily limits the body's natural cooling mechanisms, be careful not to get overheated during exercise. Wear loose-fitting, light clothing and comfortable shoes, make sure you drink enough water to avoid dehydration, and go slowly, particularly when the weather is hot or humid.

### A safe pregnancy

If you are pregnant, observe certain precautions while exercising, especially if you did not exercise regularly before

### HOW EXERCISE BENEFITS A PREGNANT WOMAN

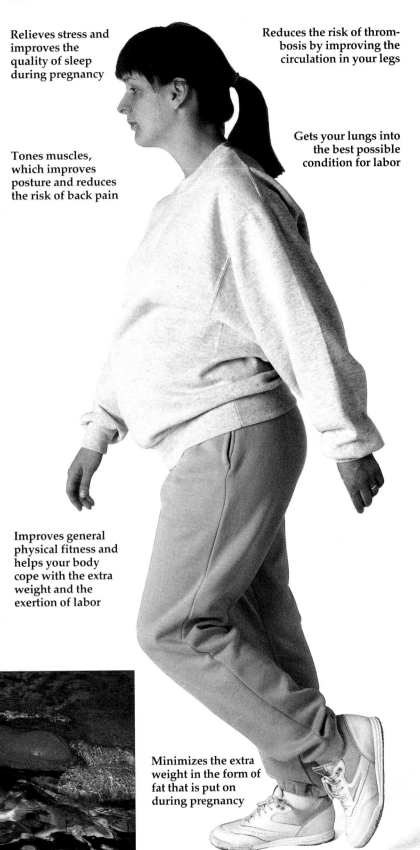

**Relieves stress and improves the quality of sleep during pregnancy**

**Reduces the risk of thrombosis by improving the circulation in your legs**

**Tones muscles, which improves posture and reduces the risk of back pain**

**Gets your lungs into the best possible condition for labor**

**Improves general physical fitness and helps your body cope with the extra weight and the exertion of labor**

**Minimizes the extra weight in the form of fat that is put on during pregnancy**

**Swimming**
*Many pregnant women enjoy swimming as their exercise of choice. Being in the water reduces the effect of gravity. However, do not swim in extremely cold water because of the increased risk of cramping.*

**Stretching in pregnancy**
*Squatting (right) and sitting in the position shown below can help you strengthen the muscles of your back and thighs and improve the flexibility of your pelvic joints in preparation for childbirth.*

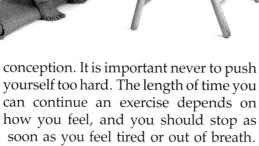

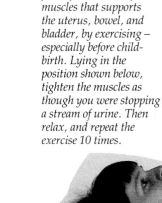

**Pelvic floor exercises**
*You can strengthen the pelvic floor, a web of muscles that supports the uterus, bowel, and bladder, by exercising – especially before childbirth. Lying in the position shown below, tighten the muscles as though you were stopping a stream of urine. Then relax, and repeat the exercise 10 times.*

conception. It is important never to push yourself too hard. The length of time you can continue an exercise depends on how you feel, and you should stop as soon as you feel tired or out of breath.

Ask your doctor to recommend an exercise program tailored for you.

Most women are able to continue some form of gentle exercise throughout their pregnancy. However, doctors prescribe complete bed rest for some women because of a possible complication. Later in your pregnancy, you may be advised to rest if your blood pressure becomes dangerously high.

The best forms of exercise during pregnancy are walking and swimming, and both can usually be continued throughout your pregnancy. Walking need not be brisk to keep you fit. Invest in a well-made pair of walking shoes with low heels. High heels encourage

arching of the lower back, which, by stretching the spinal ligaments, can cause back pain. Toward the end of your pregnancy, you may feel a dragging deep in the pelvis when you walk caused by the pressure of the baby's weight. This pressure may be eased by doing pelvic floor exercises (see below), starting early in pregnancy.

## Energetic exercise

Women accustomed to energetic exercise such as jogging or playing tennis can continue during pregnancy for as long as they feel comfortable. However, do not be surprised if you experience increased breathlessness during exertion, a loss of mobility and agility, and difficulty balancing during pregnancy because of a shift in your center of gravity.

If you did aerobic exercises before becoming pregnant, ask your doctor whether these exercises are still suitable. The increased amount of estrogen produced during pregnancy softens the ligaments and tendons that support your spine and joints, making them more vulnerable to injury. This also applies to the 6 weeks following delivery.

However experienced you are, it is not recommended that you take part in waterskiing, down-hill skiing, or horseback riding during any stage of pregnancy because of the risk of miscarriage from falling. In addition, avoid contact sports.

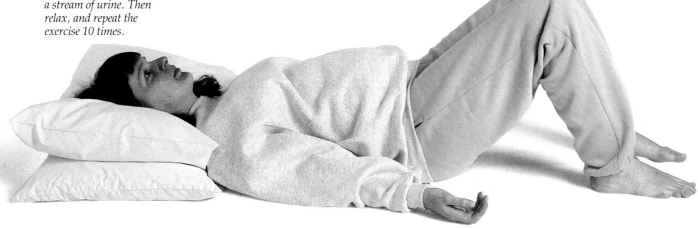

## EXERCISING AFTER CHILDBIRTH

Exercising every day can help you regain a trim appearance after your child is born. Be sure to build up slowly, and always stop if you feel pain. If you had a cesarean section, ask your doctor when it would be safe to begin exercising.

### Shoulder stretches

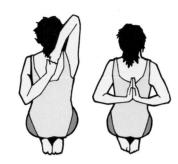

**1** Sitting on your heels, clasp your hands behind your back as shown. Hold, and repeat with your other arm raised.

**2** Put your hands behind you, palms together. As you bring your elbows back, breathe deeply.

### Strengthening muscles

Bend forward from the hips. Breathe deeply and, as you breathe out, pull in your stomach muscles. At the same time, squeeze your pelvic floor muscles. Then relax as you breathe in again.

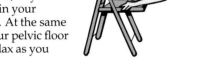

**1** Lie flat on your back with your knees bent.

**2** Breathe in, then lift your hips as you breathe out. Hold the position for a few seconds, then breathe in and bring your hips down.

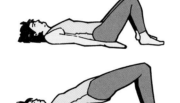

**1** Kneel on a thick rug or pad, resting on your heels. Turn your palms outward and stretch your arms above your head.

**2** Bring your arms down close to your thighs and, breathing out, fold your body forward. Lower your head until it touches the floor. Breathe naturally for about a minute. Then breathe in and straighten to an upright position while still kneeling.

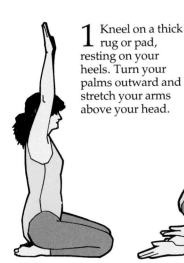

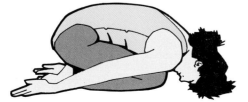

## EXERCISE AND AGING

Regular exercise can slow down the natural stiffening associated with the aging of your muscles, tendons, ligaments, bones, and joints. Exercise also helps keep your joints mobile as you age, and it reduces your risk of a serious injury from falling by maintaining your muscle strength, balance, and coordination.

### Never too late to start

There is plenty of truth in the saying that you're only as old as you feel. Today, many people view retirement not as automatic membership in the ranks of the aging, but as an opportunity to pursue new interests. The average life expectancy in the US has been steadily increasing, reaching 75 years in 1988. Current medical thinking stresses the importance of physical fitness as a part of preventive medicine for all ages.

If you are in your 60s or 70s and have never done much exercise before, you may think it is too late to start now. But it is never too late to begin enjoying the health benefits of regular exercise, as long as you use common sense.

### Estimating your fitness level

Before you can set your target level of fitness, you may need to determine how fit – or unfit – you are today. It would be dangerous to take up jogging suddenly if you have not done even moderate exercise for years and if climbing the stairs leaves you puffing for breath.

The simplest way to determine your level of physical fitness is to examine the response of your heart to exercise. If you are out of condition, your heart will beat very fast when you exercise, resulting in a rapid pulse, in order to pump more blood to your muscles. This helps supply the muscles with the additional energy they need to work harder. By contrast, if your heart is in good shape, it will not beat as rapidly because it can pump more blood with each beat.

## Knowing when to rest

If you have been inactive for a few years, or even months, talk to your doctor and then start exercising again with caution. Allow for the fact that, as you get older, it will take you longer to bounce back to normal after exercise and to recover from an injury. If your heart begins to race – stop, rest, and wait until it slows down before starting again. People who are seriously out of shape may have to stop frequently. Gradually, as your level of physical fitness improves, you will be able to exercise for longer periods without resting. Although your ultimate goal should be to exercise with few rests, never force yourself to continue if you don't feel right. Working your body too hard when you are not sufficiently fit can be extremely dangerous.

## Setting your own pace

The best type of exercise is one that fits easily into your everyday life, such as cycling to the stores, climbing the stairs rather than taking the elevator, working in the backyard, or walking to the park.

Exercises for older people should never be physically punishing. Try to exercise at least three or four times a week, and remember to increase the length of your exercise sessions very gradually. Once you have reached your desired level of fitness, continue exercising regularly to ensure that you stay in shape.

## WARMING UP BEFORE EXERCISE

Whatever form of exercise you choose, it is always wise (especially when you are older) to spend a few minutes loosening up your joints and muscles before beginning.

**Arm swings**
*Stand with your feet 1 foot apart and swing your right arm forward and then backward. Repeat with your left arm. Repeat 5 times.*

**Body bends**
*Stand with your feet 1 foot apart and put your hands on your hips. Lean forward slowly, bending as far as you can comfortably manage; then bend backward. Repeat 5 times.*

**Body stretches**
*Stand with your feet 1 foot apart. Place both hands over your head and lean gently to one side of your body, as shown. Repeat slowly on the other side. Repeat 5 times on each side.*

---

**WARNING**

Older people should limit their exercise if it aggravates arthritis or causes pain or pressure in the chest, dizziness, palpitations, severe breathlessness, or extreme fatigue. If you have heart trouble or any symptom mentioned above, consult your doctor.

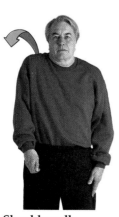

**Shoulder rolls**
*With your feet 1 foot apart, roll one shoulder forward, then backward, 5 times for each shoulder.*

# CASE HISTORY
# NERVOUS ABOUT RETIREMENT

**P**ETER IS SCHEDULED TO RETIRE **in a few months and is depressed at the prospect. He is used to a busy and active life at work, and the idea of the empty days stretching out before him seems upsetting. Peter decides to consult a personnel counselor at his company who advises employees on retirement.**

**PERSONAL DETAILS**
**Name** Peter Kowalski
**Age** 65
**Occupation** Engineer
**Family** Peter is married to Eva, who is a year older than he is and works full-time running her own business.

## BACKGROUND
Peter has worked for the same company for more than 30 years and has been promoted from junior assistant to chief engineer in one of the biggest shipping companies in the US. He is good at his job and enjoys its challenges, as well as the social stimulation of working in a large organization. Although he has a white-collar job, he has kept active visiting his company's many plants.

## THE CONSULTATION
The counselor asks Peter what he plans to do when he retires, and Peter confesses that he has not given it a great deal of thought. He talks vaguely about having time to read more, and how he has always planned to do more around the house when he has the time.

The counselor asks Peter whether he is involved in any form of physical activity in his leisure time. Peter says that he greatly enjoyed sports when he was younger, and occasionally he has worked out in a gym subsidized by his company.

## THE INTERPRETATION
The counselor realizes that Peter is worried about his upcoming retirement. This is because Peter fears that the end of his working life signals the beginning of old age. The counselor tells Peter that many people launch themselves into new and challenging phases of their lives well into their 70s. Many marathon runners who have been active over the years are over age 65. He reminds Peter that it is important to remain physically fit, mentally alert, and active even when he is retired.

## THE ADVICE
Peter's counselor advises him to join a health club, where he will be able to get regular exercise in a social setting. The counselor also suggests taking classes in subjects of interest. He mentions that hobbies, community service, or volunteer work could all help make retirement worthwhile and fulfilling.

## THE OUTLOOK
Peter agrees to consider his counselor's advice. Peter and Eva discuss the importance of enjoying retirement. They both decide to join the local park district where Peter becomes involved in a program to help the homeless. Also, Eva and Peter swim at the park at least three times a week and they have joined the local senior citizens' group. Peter's mental health and physical fitness both improve and, as a result, he thrives during his retirement.

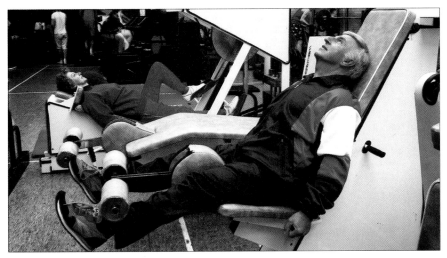

**Health clubs**
*A health club provides opportunities for physical exercise and social interchange.*

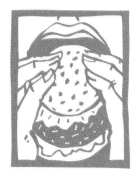

# EXERCISE AND BEING OVERWEIGHT

**M**OST PEOPLE BECOME overweight because they take in more energy in their food than they expend during physical activity and other metabolic processes. If you are overweight and want to lose weight, you may not find it easy to do so only by cutting calories. It may also be necessary to increase the amount of energy you use, and the best way to do this is to exercise more.

One disadvantage of being overweight is that your skeletal frame must carry a greater load (although many overweight women have stronger than average bones). This increases the strain on the joints of your spine, hips, knees, and ankles, which, in turn, increases the likelihood of injury and of aggravating any arthritis in your weight-bearing joints. Overweight people tend to exercise less than those of normal weight, and they become breathless more quickly and are generally less physically fit.

**Dietary choices**
*Always look for low-calorie alternatives when you are buying food. As a dessert, fruit is less fattening than an ice cream sundae.*

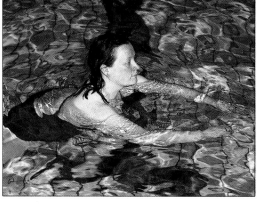

**Swimming**
*Swimming is a particularly good exercise if you are overweight because the water supports your weight while you exercise many different muscle groups.*

## LOW-INTENSITY EXERCISE

The body relies mainly on two sources of fuel for energy – carbohydrates and fat. Contrary to what many people believe, more fat is burned during low-intensity exercise. In addition, the longer you exercise, the higher the proportion of fat burned by the body.

The value of exercise in losing weight is in the amount of energy you expend in relation to the calories you consume in your diet. The key to exercising for weight loss is to select an exercise you enjoy and will continue to do regularly. If you are markedly overweight, get advice from your doctor before beginning an exercise program.

### Pre-aerobic activities

When you are overweight, start exercising with "pre-aerobic" activities. These are aerobic in nature but are at a lower level of intensity than the strenuous activity needed for aerobic fitness.

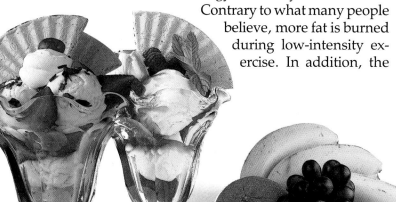

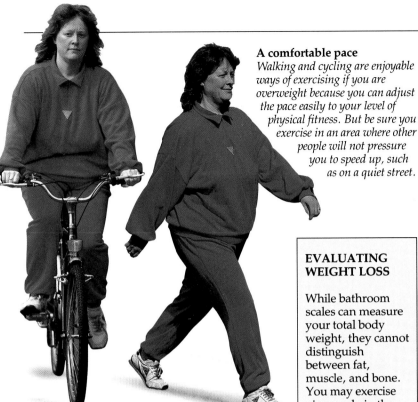

**A comfortable pace**
*Walking and cycling are enjoyable ways of exercising if you are overweight because you can adjust the pace easily to your level of physical fitness. But be sure you exercise in an area where other people will not pressure you to speed up, such as on a quiet street.*

Pre-aerobic activities are a good way to exercise for weight loss, though they are not strenuous enough to improve your fitness unless you do them regularly for a long period of time. They will, however, help strengthen your bones, ligaments, tendons, and joints.

## Getting started
Pre-aerobic activities include walking, cycling, and swimming, all at a moderate pace. It is a good idea to try a variety of activities. This allows you to rest different parts of your body, avoiding the risk of injury, as well as reducing any boredom you feel from a single activity.

It is best to build up gradually, starting with 5 to 10 minutes a session. Providing you do not experience persistent aches and pains, you can eventually increase your exercise time to between 40 minutes and 1 hour per session.

Try exercising like this three or four times a week for the first few weeks of a weight-loss diet. Then, when you have lost weight, you can concentrate on raising your level of physical fitness by building up to daily moderate exercise.

---

### EVALUATING WEIGHT LOSS

While bathroom scales can measure your total body weight, they cannot distinguish between fat, muscle, and bone. You may exercise vigorously in the hope of losing weight and be disappointed to find that you have not lost much weight. But you may be pleasantly surprised to find that your clothes fit better than before. The explanation is simple. As a result of exercising, you lost fat but gained muscle, a distinction not revealed by the bathroom scales. Also, your body will become less flabby as you tone your muscles through exercise. To lose weight, you must cut down on the calories you take in as well as increase your level of physical activity.

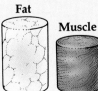

**Fat**

**Muscle**

---

## ASK YOUR DOCTOR
### EXERCISE AND BEING OVERWEIGHT

**Q** If I have been exercising regularly and then stop, will my muscle turn into fat?

**A** Fat and muscle are two different kinds of tissue, so it is not possible for one to turn into the other. If, however, you stop exercising while maintaining the same calorie intake, your muscles will weaken and diminish in size, and the excess calories will be stored as fat. So, although it is not possible for muscle literally to turn into fat, this may seem to be what happens.

**Q** I'm very overweight and I need more exercise. But all exercise seems to do is make me hungrier, so I end up eating more. Is there any way out of this vicious circle?

**A** Yes – eat sensibly. If you are hungry, eat foods from the fruit, vegetable, and high-fiber groups that are low in calories. Avoid desserts and snacks that contain many calories.

**Q** I'm 60 years old, physically fit, and hoping to lose weight. My wife says I should go jogging, but I'm worried that this could damage my joints or bones. Am I right?

**A** Do not jog without your doctor's approval especially if you have any heart disease. However, as long as your joints are fairly flexible, regular exercise may postpone the development of joint problems. Begin by walking briskly and gradually increase the distance to work up to jogging. You may find that regular walking sessions will help you lose weight and that you don't need to take up running.

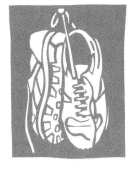

# EXERCISE AND SICKNESS

**E**XERCISE IS NOT JUST for healthy people. Although there are some people with medical disorders for whom exercise is not recommended, in most cases it is important to stay as active as possible. People who think of themselves as invalids and don't perform any exercise are likely to have greater problems; they may experience a steady deterioration in their health.

If you have a medical problem and want to start an exercise program, you should first consult your doctor and discuss the type of activities that he or she believes are safe for you. The following sections offer some useful general information about exercising if you have one of a variety of common medical conditions.

## WHAT CONDITIONS CAN EXERCISE IMPROVE?

Regular exercise can actually ease or slow the progression of certain disorders or conditions, reducing your risk of complications and helping you remain more mobile and independent.

**How swimming can help relieve back pain**
*Swimming helps strengthen the back and abdominal muscles that support your spine. Being immersed in water reduces the effects of the force of gravity, so swimming movements do not place undue stress on your back.*

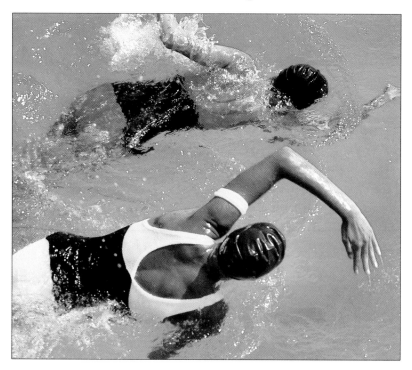

## Back pain

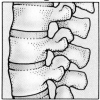

A recent study showed that people with chronic recurrent back pain who participate in some form of regular exercise manage the pain better than those who remain inactive. Before you decide to do any particular type of exercise, consult your doctor about the cause of your back pain. If you have osteoporosis or problems with vertebral discs, a doctor should guide you in your exercise program. But much back pain is caused by muscle spasms and does not have a specific cause. Swimming may be the best type of exercise for anyone with back pain. When you swim the breaststroke, you should be sure you put your face in the water every few strokes. If you keep your head out of the water all the time, you will be arching your lower back, and that movement, by stretching the spinal ligaments, is likely to aggravate your back pain.

If you are a jogger with chronic or recurrent back pain, avoid hard surfaces and wear cushioned insoles to reduce the amount of jarring through the spine each time your feet strike the ground.

If you have had back or disc problems, it is also important to take extra care when you do any strength exercises that involve lifting weights. Use an exercise mat for any floor exercises that you do, and always keep your knees bent (not straight) during a sit-up routine to reduce the chances of injury to your lower back.

# HOW EXERCISING CAN HELP HEART CONDITIONS

In the past, people with heart conditions were advised to rest since doctors thought that vigorous exercise could make the condition worse. However, studies have now shown that, as long as you follow basic safety rules, exercising is safe and can help improve selected conditions. Ask your doctor for some guidelines before you begin exercising.

### Angina and heart attacks

Angina is chest pain that is usually brought on by exercise or stress and is relieved by rest and relaxation. Angina is caused by an insufficient supply of oxygen to the heart muscle, which in turn is usually caused by narrowed coronary arteries (see illustration). Gentle exercise is good for most people with angina because it improves their fitness and their spirits.

Like angina, a heart attack is a result of coronary heart disease. A heart attack occurs when an artery becomes blocked by a blood clot, which leads to death of the area of the heart muscle the artery supplies. It takes about 6 weeks for the surrounding damaged heart muscle to heal. Thereafter, most people can benefit from a program of regular aerobic exercise under a doctor's care. Exercise improves your blood flow, or circulation, and may reduce your chances of having another heart attack.

### How exercise helps a failing heart

A recent study has shown that a program of aerobic exercise can improve the pumping efficiency of the heart and thus help reduce symptoms of heart failure such as breathlessness and edema (swelling) of the ankles.

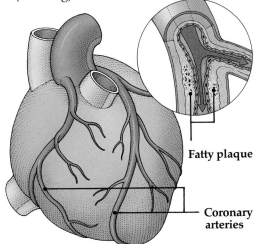

**Fatty plaque**

**Coronary arteries**

**EXERCISING SAFELY WITH A HEART CONDITION**

◆ Gradually build up the effort you make and the time you spend over several weeks.
◆ Avoid exercising in very cold or very hot weather, or right after a meal.
◆ Avoid lifting heavy loads or doing strenuous exercise.
◆ Stop if any of the warning signs of heart problems begin to develop (see WARNING below).

**Coronary heart disease**
*In coronary heart disease, blood flow through the coronary arteries slows down when an artery becomes narrowed by deposits of fatty plaque on the artery walls.*

## Arthritis

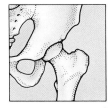

Exercise is good for most people with arthritis because it helps keep the joints mobile and the surrounding muscles, tendons, and ligaments strong. You will know if you are doing too much exercise or the wrong type if any of your joints become stiffer, more painful, or more swollen.

Swimming and cycling are more suitable than running if you have arthritis, because these activities do not involve putting your full weight on the joints of your hips, knees, ankles, and feet. If you exercise outdoors in cold weather, make sure that you wear warm socks and gloves; this helps prevent stiffness.

## High blood pressure

Regular aerobic activities are usually recommended for people with hypertension. Exercise can help you reduce your blood pressure. There is a controversy, however, over whether anyone with high blood pressure should avoid the strain of isometric strength training and lifting heavy weights.

Some drugs (known as beta blockers) that are used to lower blood pressure suppress the response of the heart to strenuous exercise. If you are taking a beta blocker (such as acebutolol or propranolol), remember that you will not be able to accurately gauge your condition during exertion by checking your pulse.

**WARNING**

Stop exercising immediately if you have any of the following heart symptoms:

◆ chest pain
◆ pain spreading to the neck, jaw, or arms (especially the left arm)
◆ palpitations
◆ dizziness
◆ nausea or indigestion
◆ blurred vision
◆ light-headedness
◆ severe breathlessness
◆ feeling faint or fainting

## VARICOSE VEINS

If you have varicose veins, physical activity that exercises your legs can help reduce discomfort and swelling by improving the circulation of blood through your veins. But if you find that walking or running causes more pain in your veins and legs, try wearing elastic support hose. If they don't help, take up an alternative activity such as swimming. Anyone with varicose veins who takes part in vigorous exercise should wear elastic support hose to minimize the congestion of blood in veins and the resulting accumulation in muscles.

## Diabetes

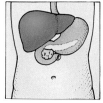

Regular daily exercise is important for the control of diabetes and may help reduce the dose of insulin or the dose of oral medication taken by people who are not dependent on insulin. If you are a diabetic taking medication, you may need to increase your intake of carbohydrates before you exercise. Check with your doctor on how to adjust your diet and medication in relation to regular physical activity.

All diabetics should carry a supply of sugar or candy in case exercise induces hypoglycemia, a sudden drop in blood sugar that may cause dizziness, sweating, nausea, or a loss of concentration. If you don't quickly eat or drink some sweet food or liquid, you may collapse and lose consciousness.

You should tell the people with whom you exercise that you are diabetic, in case you have an episode of hypoglycemia. This is especially important if your diabetes has not been stabilized yet and your blood sugar level is apt to fall unpredictably. If a diabetic does become unconscious from hypoglycemia, medical help should be summoned immediately; the doctor will give an injection of glucose or of the hormone glucagon, which raises the blood sugar level.

**Exercising with diabetes**
*If you have diabetes, you may need to drink a sweet liquid or eat a food containing sugar just before you exercise. You should also carry sugar or candy with you in case your blood sugar level drops.*

## Stroke

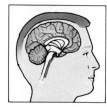

A program of exercises after a stroke can help the patient regain the use of muscles and joints and restore independence and mobility. Depending on the degree of paralysis from the stroke, these exercises may include passive movements, in which someone physically moves your arms and legs for you, or active movements that you initiate yourself. You may also spend time in a heated swimming pool, where you will find each movement easier to perform because the water supports the weight of your body.

If you recover enough to be able to stand and take a few steps, you will learn to walk again, at first with assistance and then using a walker or cane.

Once you are ready to be discharged from the hospital, you and your caregiver will need to learn a range of exercises for you to do at home to help continue your recovery. The more active you are, the better your prospects are for rehabilitation to an independent life-style.

## Peripheral vascular disease

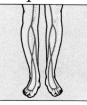

Peripheral vascular disease is a condition in which the blood flow through the arteries, primarily in the legs, is impaired. As a result, the muscles are deprived of oxygen during exercise, causing cramps. Exertion causes pain in the muscles of your legs that becomes more severe, until you have to stop moving and rest for a few moments. After a short rest, you may be able to continue moving or walking.

Recent studies have shown that people with this condition who try to exercise regularly despite pain are able to steadily increase the distance they can walk, but those who rest as soon as the discomfort begins are more likely to have serious problems.

## SHOULD I EXERCISE IF I HAVE OTHER DISORDERS?

Exercise does not always help ease the symptoms of a disease or condition. However, even those who have a disorder not necessarily helped by exercise (like those in this section) should do as much as they can comfortably, for the good of their overall health.

### Asthma

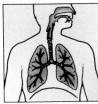

If you have asthma and find that exercise brings on symptoms such as breathlessness, wheezing, coughing, or tightness across the chest, try inhaling a dose of your bronchodilator a few minutes before you begin to exercise next time. Your doctor may also describe other steps that could be effective in preventing an attack.

Some people who have asthma find that they can cope better with certain types of physical activity, such as prolonged moderate exercise. Swimming in an indoor pool where the air is warm and humid is one example. You may also consider jogging slowly or taking up a sport that involves intermittent bouts of exertion. A few asthmatics compete in long-distance races such as marathons, but this requires special conditioning.

Because cold air often precipitates an attack of asthma, it is smart to wear a scarf across your nose or mouth when you walk or jog in cold weather.

### TOP ATHLETES WITH ASTHMA

A number of athletes are able to perform extremely well despite their asthma. These athletes must be careful not to take any drug for their condition that would eliminate them from competition, but most asthma medication is acceptable to sports authorities.

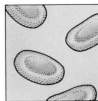

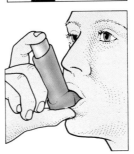

**Exercising with asthma**
*If you have asthma and discover that exercise brings on your symptoms, you may find it helpful to use an inhaler (above) before you start.*

### Parkinson's disease

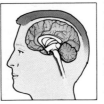

Parkinson's disease is a brain disorder that causes shaking, weakness, and stiffness. These symptoms gradually become more severe the longer you have this disease.

It is important for anyone with Parkinson's disease to remain as active as possible, perhaps by walking or doing some light gardening or housework. Regular warm-up exercises that get the muscles working and keep the joints moving may improve your posture and help you stay independent and mobile.

Even in severe cases, when you are no longer able to move around without assistance, passive exercises, in which someone else moves different parts of your body for you, can help minimize muscle weakness and joint stiffness.

## WHEN IS IT DANGEROUS TO EXERCISE?

With the following diseases or disorders, you should not exercise until the condition has been treated. For some diagnoses you need to take special care to avoid doing further damage to your health.

### Anemia

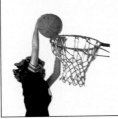

In anemia the amount of hemoglobin, the oxygen-carrying pigment in the red blood cells, is reduced. Symptoms such as fatigue, breathlessness, and dizziness are caused by the decreased concentrations of hemoglobin, which delivers oxygen around the body. These symptoms become more severe during exercise. If you have anemia, the amount of exercise you do will in large part be limited by the diminished oxygen-carrying capacity of the decreased number of red blood cells.

Anemia definitely causes symptoms when hemoglobin levels fall below 8

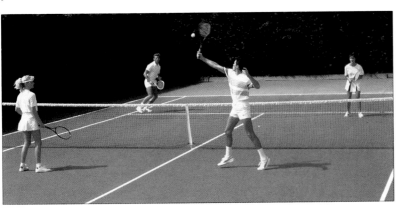

grams per 100 milliliters (normal levels are 14 to 16 grams per 100 milliliters for men and 12 to 14 grams per 100 milliliters for women). However, symptoms develop in some people when hemoglobin levels are still around 10 grams per 100 milliliters. Other reasons for the anemia may exist. However, this may be the result of an iron deficiency. Results of blood tests may reveal depleted iron stores but symptoms rapidly improve when the cause of anemia is discovered and treated.

People with symptoms of anemia should see a doctor to confirm the diagnosis and to establish how severe the disease is and what the cause might be. In the meantime, those with symptoms of anemia should rest until the problem has been corrected. Exercise can be resumed once the level of hemoglobin in the blood is almost back to normal and the person with anemia is symptom-free, both at rest and during exertion.

## Infection

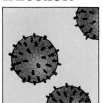 If you have symptoms of an infection, such as a fever, a cough that produces phlegm, a sore throat, or swollen glands, you should not participate in any form of strenuous exercise. Not only is your performance likely to be impaired, but any overexertion is highly likely to make your infection worse and to delay recovery.

This "no exercise" rule should be applied to all types of acute infection including influenza, bronchitis, pneumonia, and cystitis. Exercise can facilitate the spread of the infection into the bloodstream and to other organs.

It is important for anyone with symptoms of a viral infection to rest, at least at home if not in bed. Vigorous exercise may lead to inflammation of vital organs such as the liver (hepatitis) or heart (myocarditis).

## Epilepsy

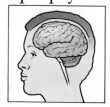 If you have epilepsy and your condition is well controlled by medication, you should be able to take part in most forms of exercise. However, because symptoms often occur without warning, always make sure that you exercise only when someone else is present to help you if you have an attack. In particular, people with epilepsy should never swim unaccompanied, to prevent drowning.

It is also important for epileptics to ensure they eat and drink sufficient amounts of food and liquids before exercising because hypoglycemia (a drop in blood sugar) and dehydration can both provoke a seizure.

Some sports are dangerous for people with epilepsy. Football carries risks of damage to brain tissue from a blow to the head. Wear protective headgear when you participate in any contact sport.

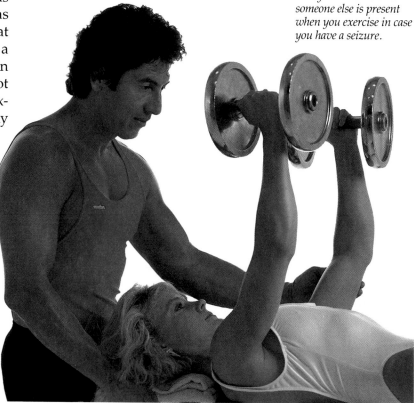

**WARNING**

Many people who exercise regularly are tempted to continue their regular exercise routine even when they are not feeling well. However, when you have an infection, exercise can make your condition worse. Do not exercise if you have any of the following symptoms of infection:

♦ fever
♦ sore throat
♦ swollen glands
♦ cough that produces phlegm
♦ genital discharge
♦ painful urination.

**Exercising with epilepsy**
*If you have epilepsy, always make sure that someone else is present when you exercise in case you have a seizure.*

# CASE HISTORY
# MUSCLE WEAKNESS

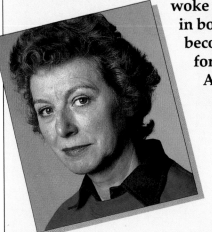

**A**RLENE HAD THE FLU during a recent outbreak, but it has now been 3 weeks since she first fell ill. Although the sore throat, fever, and muscle pains have gone, she still feels very tired and this morning she woke with numbness and tingling in both legs. Her legs have also become weak, making it difficult for her to walk. Alarmed, Arlene called her doctor.

**PERSONAL DETAILS**
**Name** Arlene Ruggiero
**Age** 44
**Occupation** Swimming coach
**Family** Arlene is adopted and does not know anything about her birth parents' medical history. Her adoptive parents are healthy.

## MEDICAL BACKGROUND
Arlene has not seen a doctor for several years. Her job makes it easy for her to stay in shape by swimming.

## THE CONSULTATION
Arlene describes the symptoms to her doctor. The weakness in her legs has become worse and she can hardly move her right foot. She has also started to get a pins-and-needles sensation in both hands. The doctor finds that Arlene feels nothing when she is pricked with pins anywhere below her knees. There is a possibility that Arlene has injured herself at the swimming pool, so the doctor arranges for her to be admitted immediately to the hospital.

## THE NEUROLOGIST'S CONSULTATION
The neurologist performs a lumbar puncture and sends a sample of Arlene's cerebrospinal fluid to the laboratory for analysis. Electrical tests on her legs and arms confirm that nerve impulses are not conducted normally to her muscles.

## THE DIAGNOSIS
A diagnosis of GUILLAIN-BARRÉ SYNDROME, a rare neurological disorder, is confirmed by the results of the electrical tests and a CT scan. The doctor needs the CT scan to exclude forms of central nervous system disease that produce similar symptoms. Also, the laboratory report shows an abnormal protein in Arlene's cerebrospinal fluid.

## THE TREATMENT
There is no specific treatment, but it is important for Arlene's condition to be monitored in the hospital in case she has difficulty breathing. After 6 days the pins-and-needles sensation eases and Arlene begins to regain feeling in her arms and legs. The neurologist tells her that she will need a period of rehabilitation.

At first most of the muscle exercises are passive, with the therapist moving parts of Arlene's body for her. Slowly, she begins to do the exercises herself and the strength returns to her muscles as she continues to exercise. Arlene then starts regular sessions in the hydrotherapy pool where she floats in the water and it is easier for her to move her joints through their full range of motion.

Once she returns home from the hospital, swimming provides the key to Arlene's full recovery. She swims every day, slowly building up her speed and distance. After another 3 months of visits to the pool and the gym, Arlene is as active as she was before her illness.

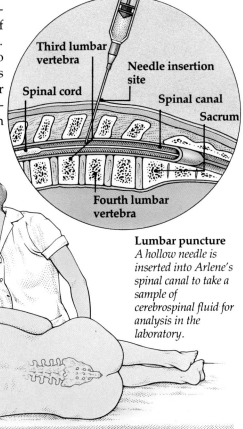

Third lumbar vertebra
Needle insertion site
Spinal cord
Spinal canal
Sacrum
Fourth lumbar vertebra

**Lumbar puncture**
*A hollow needle is inserted into Arlene's spinal canal to take a sample of cerebrospinal fluid for analysis in the laboratory.*

# CHAPTER THREE

# A GUIDE TO FITNESS

INTRODUCTION

WHAT IS FITNESS?

HOW PHYSICALLY
FIT ARE YOU?

IMPROVING YOUR
FITNESS LEVEL

FITNESS HAS BECOME fashionable. But do people know what physical fitness means? Even though there has been virtually a revolution in the way we think about fitness, most people are still unsure about what it really involves. Being physically fit does not have to mean training for hours on end in order to win awards. Physical fitness does not equal athletic excellence and, for most people, fitness and performance are two different things. For most of us, fitness means being able to meet the demands of everyday life and still have extra energy in reserve to meet sudden unexpected demands. The idea is to be able to carry a heavy shopping bag without great difficulty, not to compete as the weight lifter of the year; to enjoy a regular game of tennis, not to win the Davis cup.

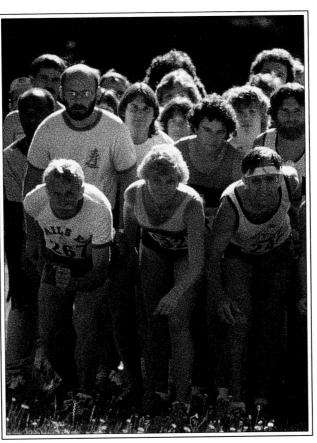

Many people have an unrealistic view of their own level of physical fitness. In this chapter we offer a definition of the three elements of fitness – strength, the ability to carry, lift, push, or pull any heavy load; flexibility, the ability to bend, stretch, and twist; and endurance, the ability to continue exercising without a break for a prolonged period. We also review the most common physical activities, including not only sports but also everyday activities such as walking, climbing stairs, and gardening. Each one is rated according to the degree of strength, flexibility, and endurance that you need to perform it.

We then ask you to determine how physically fit you are. Most people overestimate their level of physical fitness and think of themselves as being in better shape than they actually are. We encourage you to be honest with yourself and to assess your personal level of fitness realistically. You may want to ask your doctor to help you.

In this chapter, we include ways in which you can test not only your strength, flexibility, and endurance, but also the efficiency of your heart. Some of the methods people used in the past to determine their fitness levels are now considered too strenuous for people who have been inactive for a while, those who are overweight, or older people. An important message in this chapter is that moderate exercise – performed regularly– will substantially benefit your physical health (and your mental health, too).

Finally, we suggest ways in which you can improve your level of physical fitness. We offer a variety of different activities, along with recommendations on how often you should probably exercise.

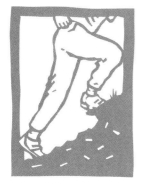

# WHAT IS FITNESS?

IN THE 1990s, the word "fitness" seems to appear often in conversation and in the media. What exactly does the word mean? Fitness is the ability to perform physical activities without becoming unduly fatigued or breathless. Your level of fitness is a reflection of how efficiently your heart and muscles can use oxygen and expend energy. And that efficiency is, in turn, primarily determined by your physical activity habits.

Many people do not honestly face up to their own level of fitness. Some do not exercise much, yet, because they are seldom sick, pride themselves on being physically fit. They confuse good health with good physical condition. Others do minimal exercise and think they are physically fit in spite of it. However, you are physically fit only if you do some type of moderate exercise at least three or four times a week.

## THE ELEMENTS OF FITNESS

Fitness involves three elements – strength, flexibility, and endurance. You may want to consider your exercise program or favorite sport in relation to these elements by using the box on the opposite page. Because each activity places different demands on your strength, flexibility, and endurance, it is important

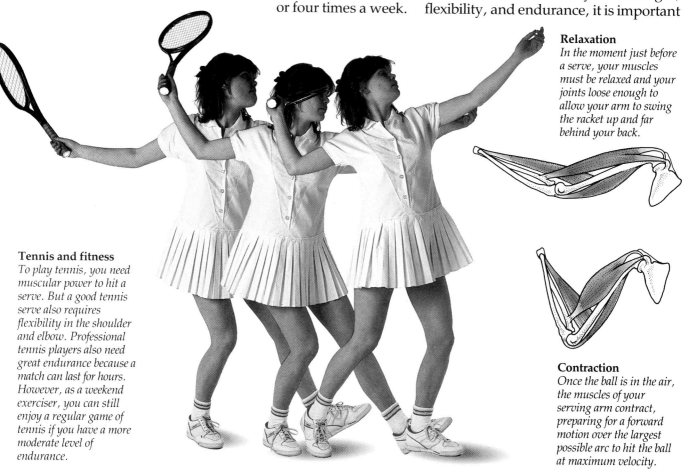

**Tennis and fitness**
*To play tennis, you need muscular power to hit a serve. But a good tennis serve also requires flexibility in the shoulder and elbow. Professional tennis players also need great endurance because a match can last for hours. However, as a weekend exerciser, you can still enjoy a regular game of tennis if you have a more moderate level of endurance.*

**Relaxation**
*In the moment just before a serve, your muscles must be relaxed and your joints loose enough to allow your arm to swing the racket up and far behind your back.*

**Contraction**
*Once the ball is in the air, the muscles of your serving arm contract, preparing for a forward motion over the largest possible arc to hit the ball at maximum velocity.*

to develop a program that benefits a maximum number of muscle groups.

## Strength

Strength is your ability to carry, lift, push, or pull any heavy load. Ideally, between one quarter and one half of your body weight should be made up of the muscle tissue that gives you strength.

There are about 400 muscles attached to your skeleton by tendons. By contracting and relaxing, your muscles control the movements of your body. However, if your muscles are out of condition, routine lifting and carrying become problems. Backache often occurs because people have allowed their back and stomach muscles to weaken, making them vulnerable to over-straining.

## Flexibility

Flexibility is your ability to bend, stretch, and twist. These movements require muscles, tendons, and joints that move easily. Flexibility is important because physical activities and sports frequently require agility and mobility. Tight leg and back muscles interfere with movement and can cause back pain and stiffness after exertion.

Supple, elastic muscles usually can absorb the shock of quick or sudden contractions, while tight ones may "pull" or tear at a critical moment and result in pain and injury. Women tend to be more flexible than men. A woman's flexibility usually peaks in her late teens or early 20s, several years before a man's, and declines very gradually.

## Endurance

Endurance is your ability to continue exercising without a break for a prolonged period. Poor endurance leads to muscle fatigue, increasing your risk of injury. It's important to understand that your heart muscle is jeopardized by exercise only if you have heart disease or anemia.

## PHYSICAL ACTIVITIES – WHICH ELEMENTS OF FITNESS DO YOU NEED?

The table below lists a range of physical activities and rates each according to the strength, flexibility, and endurance needed to perform it. The demands made by these activities depend, in part, on how vigorously you perform them.

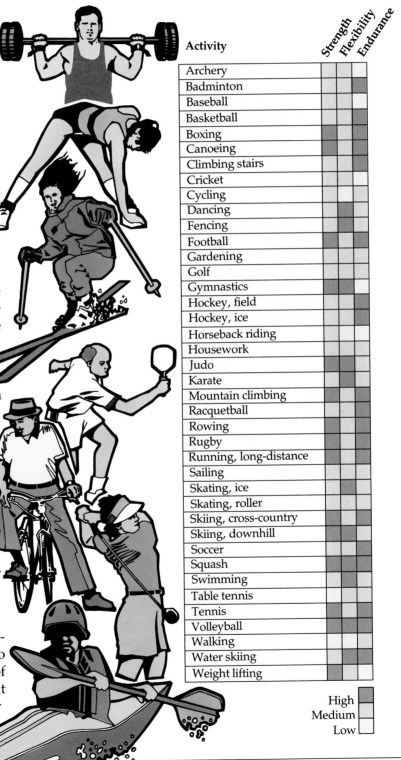

| Activity | Strength | Flexibility | Endurance |
| --- | --- | --- | --- |
| Archery | Low | Low | Medium |
| Badminton | Low | Medium | High |
| Baseball | Medium | Medium | Low |
| Basketball | Medium | Medium | High |
| Boxing | High | Medium | High |
| Canoeing | High | Medium | High |
| Climbing stairs | Medium | Low | High |
| Cricket | Medium | Medium | Low |
| Cycling | Medium | Low | High |
| Dancing | Low | High | Medium |
| Fencing | Medium | High | Medium |
| Football | High | Medium | Medium |
| Gardening | Medium | Medium | Low |
| Golf | Low | Medium | Low |
| Gymnastics | High | High | Medium |
| Hockey, field | Medium | Medium | High |
| Hockey, ice | Medium | Medium | High |
| Horseback riding | Medium | Medium | Medium |
| Housework | Low | Medium | Low |
| Judo | High | High | Medium |
| Karate | High | High | Medium |
| Mountain climbing | High | Medium | High |
| Racquetball | Medium | High | High |
| Rowing | High | Medium | High |
| Rugby | High | Medium | High |
| Running, long-distance | Medium | Low | High |
| Sailing | Medium | Medium | Low |
| Skating, ice | Medium | High | Medium |
| Skating, roller | Medium | Medium | Medium |
| Skiing, cross-country | High | Medium | High |
| Skiing, downhill | High | Medium | Medium |
| Soccer | Medium | Medium | High |
| Squash | Medium | High | High |
| Swimming | Medium | High | High |
| Table tennis | Low | Medium | Medium |
| Tennis | Medium | High | Medium |
| Volleyball | Medium | Medium | Medium |
| Walking | Low | Low | Medium |
| Water skiing | High | Medium | Medium |
| Weight lifting | High | Low | Low |

High
Medium
Low

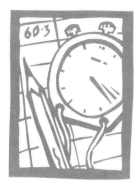

# HOW PHYSICALLY FIT ARE YOU?

**I**F YOU ARE ABOUT to start an exercise program, first assess your level of fitness. Tests that are monitored in an exercise physiology laboratory provide the most accurate results, but there are also several simple tests you can do yourself to get a general idea of your strength, flexibility, and endurance. You may want to repeat these tests periodically to help you monitor your improvement.

The most scientific method of assessing your personal endurance is the measurement of your maximum oxygen consumption, or $VO_2$ max. This is the volume of oxygen you are able to use when you exercise to your maximum capacity. However, a $VO_2$ max test takes a lot of time and requires complex equipment and the services of a staff trained in the science of exercise physiology.

## SELF-ASSESSMENT

You can easily assess your fitness level by seeing how well you do at different activities. If you gasp for breath after climbing a flight of stairs, your heart and lungs are probably out of shape. The following self-assessment program will help you evaluate your condition.

## TESTING YOUR STRENGTH

One method of measuring muscle strength is to see how many sit-ups you can do in 60 seconds. Lie on your back with your knees bent and anchor your ankles under a solid object or ask someone to hold them in position. Clasp your hands behind your head; then, using your abdominal muscles, pull yourself up to a sitting position, raising your head first and then raising your shoulders. It is essential to keep your knees bent; otherwise, you may strain your lower back. About 20 to 25 sit-ups in a minute is the average for people under 50. If you are out of shape, don't even try to do that many at first.

## TESTING YOUR FLEXIBILITY

To test your flexibility, you can do a sit-and-reach test. Tape a piece of string in a straight line onto the floor and then sit down with your legs slightly apart and your heels just touching the string. Keeping your knees and back straight, lean forward slowly from your waist to reach as far as you can. Measure the distance between the point you were able to reach and the string. You should be able to touch the string or get close to it. If your flexibility is limited because of tightness in your back or in your hamstring muscles, the exercises described on page 24 will help.

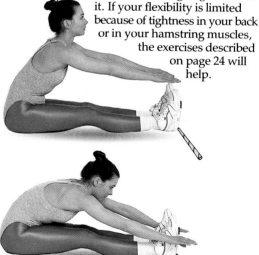

## TESTING YOUR ENDURANCE

A simple test of your endurance is to walk briskly or jog slowly for 1 mile. If you cannot complete a mile without becoming breathless or tired, your level of endurance is poor.

# TESTING THE EFFICIENCY OF YOUR HEART

The condition of your heart is a reliable indicator of your physical fitness in general. By performing the simple procedures below, you can assess the physical fitness of your heart and set objectives that can be achieved through regular exercise.

## YOUR RESTING PULSE

You can get a general idea of your endurance level by taking your pulse when you first wake in the morning – this is your resting pulse. The easiest place to feel for it is at your wrist on the side near your thumb; use the tips of your fingers. Count the number of beats over a 10-second period; then multiply by 6.

### Interpreting your result
If your resting pulse is more than 100 beats per minute, consult your doctor. Between 80 and 100 may mean that you are out of shape. About 80 beats per minute is average. Less than 70 beats per minute is usually a sign that you are physically fit. Some athletes in top condition have a resting pulse as low as 40.

### Your objective
Exercise regularly (several times a week). In time, your efforts will be rewarded by a noticeable slowing of your resting pulse.

## YOUR PULSE RECOVERY TIME

The time that it takes for your pulse to return to its normal resting rate after a period of strenuous exercise is another indicator of your fitness level.

### Interpreting your result
Depending on how vigorous the exercise is and how long you do it, this recovery time can be less than 1 minute in someone who is extremely fit. The average time is about 4 to 5 minutes, depending on your age.

### Your objective
Once you are exercising regularly you will probably find that your pulse recovery time decreases.

## YOUR TARGET HEART RATE

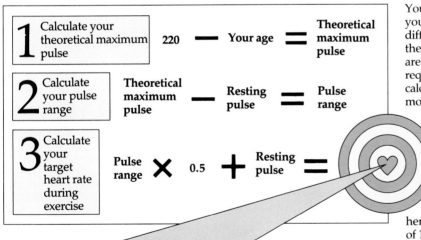

1. Calculate your theoretical maximum pulse

220 — Your age = **Theoretical maximum pulse**

2. Calculate your pulse range

**Theoretical maximum pulse** — **Resting pulse** = **Pulse range**

3. Calculate your target heart rate during exercise

**Pulse range** × 0.5 + **Resting pulse** =

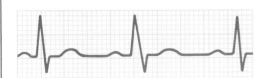

**TARGET HEART RATE DURING EXERCISE**

Your target heart rate during exercise should be your resting pulse plus about 50 percent of the difference between your resting heart rate and the theoretical maximum pulse for you. If you are seriously interested in pursuing a sport that requires great endurance, you may want to calculate your target heart rate. However, for most people, brisk walking several times a week is good exercise, and these calculations are interesting but not necessary. As an example, a woman age 50 has a resting pulse of 70. Her theoretical maximum is therefore 220 minus 50, which equals 170. Her pulse range is between 70 and 170, a difference of 100. Fifty percent of this difference (which equals 50), added to her resting pulse (70), gives a target heart rate of 120 beats per minute during exercise.

### Monitoring your pulse
After calculating your target heart rate, see how close you can get to it while you exercise. After exercising vigorously and continuously for a few minutes, count your pulse over a 10-second period. Then multiply the number by 6. Do not count your pulse for as long as a minute because your heart rate would slow down as you count.

### Your objective
To improve the efficiency of your heart, you need to exercise hard enough to achieve your target heart rate. Don't give up if you do not succeed immediately, and don't try to achieve too much in a short time.

# WALKING FOR FITNESS

Once you have established your target heart rate (see TESTING THE EFFICIENCY OF YOUR HEART on page 61) and have made the decision to get more exercise, you may want to try walking as a way of improving your physical fitness and the efficiency of your heart.

Walking is an almost ideal form of exercise, because it can fit into your daily routine, is sociable, has a low injury rate, and can be enjoyable for all ages. Walking improves your heart rate, helps you lose weight, trims your figure, and helps prevent osteoporosis. Furthermore, a large-scale study in the US has confirmed that even moderate exercise can help protect you from heart disease, cancer, and many other disorders (see page 63).

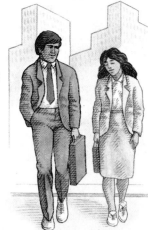

**Walking opportunities**
*The main appeal of walking is that almost everyone can do it, anywhere, and at any time. Give some thought to taking advantage of any opportunities for a brisk walk that arise in the course of a day. Sometimes you can walk to work, rather than drive or commute. Or you can walk to your train station. Leave the car at home if you need to mail a letter. Walk your children to school so that they get exercise too.*

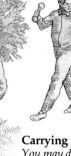

**Carrying weights**
*You may decide to wear hand and ankle weights as you walk to strengthen specific muscles and to improve circulation by making your heart work faster. For example, if you walk carrying hand weights of up to 3 pounds and use vigorous arm movements, you can strengthen the muscles in your arms and shoulders.*

## YOUR WALKING PROGRAM

Even if you have not done much exercise in the past, you are probably already in good enough shape to take a brisk walk several times a week. Start slowly, at about 2.5 to 3.5 miles per hour, and gradually build up the distance you walk. Your walking program should be enjoyable, consistent, and lifelong. A reasonable goal would be to walk for 30 to 45 minutes, at about 3 to 4 miles per hour, at least three to four times a week.

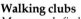

**Walking clubs**
*Many people find that they are more motivated to walk regularly if they join a walking club. Many clubs cater specifically to senior citizens. You can contact your local park district, senior center, or newspaper for names and addresses of a walking club near you.*

**Race walking**
*If you are interested in walking competitively, you may choose to enter an organized race-walking event.*

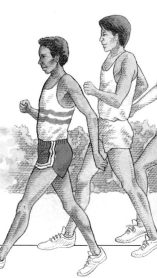

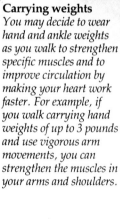

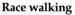

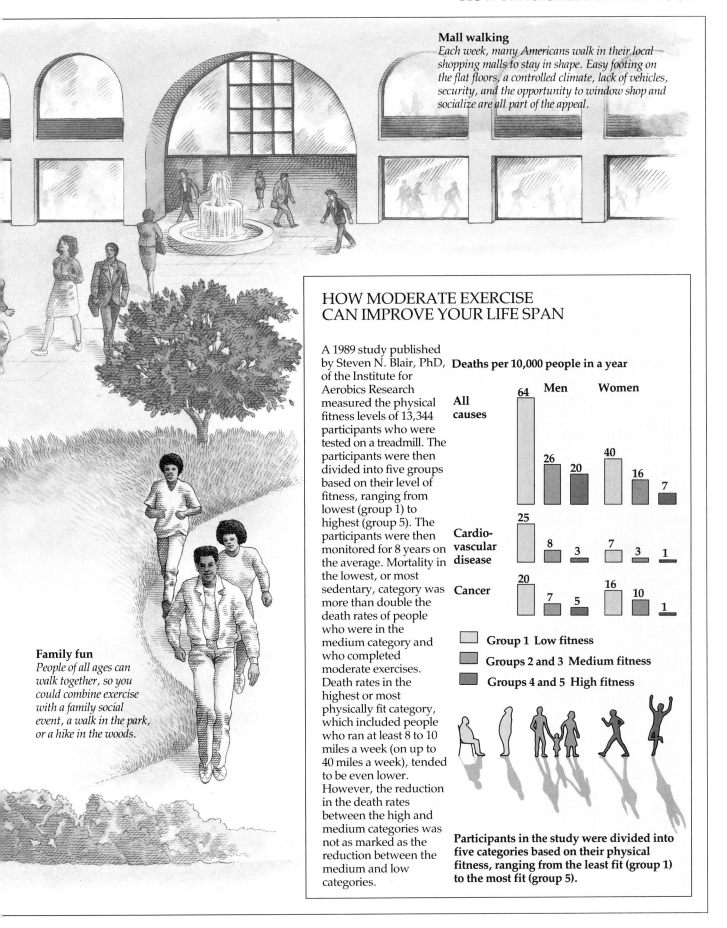

**Mall walking**
*Each week, many Americans walk in their local shopping malls to stay in shape. Easy footing on the flat floors, a controlled climate, lack of vehicles, security, and the opportunity to window shop and socialize are all part of the appeal.*

**Family fun**
*People of all ages can walk together, so you could combine exercise with a family social event, a walk in the park, or a hike in the woods.*

## HOW MODERATE EXERCISE CAN IMPROVE YOUR LIFE SPAN

A 1989 study published by Steven N. Blair, PhD, of the Institute for Aerobics Research measured the physical fitness levels of 13,344 participants who were tested on a treadmill. The participants were then divided into five groups based on their level of fitness, ranging from lowest (group 1) to highest (group 5). The participants were then monitored for 8 years on the average. Mortality in the lowest, or most sedentary, category was more than double the death rates of people who were in the medium category and who completed moderate exercises. Death rates in the highest or most physically fit category, which included people who ran at least 8 to 10 miles a week (on up to 40 miles a week), tended to be even lower. However, the reduction in the death rates between the high and medium categories was not as marked as the reduction between the medium and low categories.

**Deaths per 10,000 people in a year**

|  | Men | | Women | |
|---|---|---|---|---|
| **All causes** | 64 | 26 20 | 40 16 | 7 |
| **Cardio-vascular disease** | 25 | 8 3 | 7 3 | 1 |
| **Cancer** | 20 | 7 5 | 16 10 | 1 |

Group 1  Low fitness

Groups 2 and 3  Medium fitness

Groups 4 and 5  High fitness

**Participants in the study were divided into five categories based on their physical fitness, ranging from the least fit (group 1) to the most fit (group 5).**

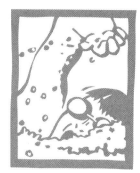

# IMPROVING YOUR FITNESS LEVEL

**W**HETHER YOU ARE a first-rate athlete training for the Olympics or an average person who just wants to get in shape, your exercise routine should include aerobic exercises, muscle-strengthening exercises, and flexibility exercises. The main difference between athletes and beginners is the amount of time and effort put into building or improving physical condition.

Baseball players not only practice their batting or pitching, they also run, skip rope, or cycle to improve their endurance, and sometimes lift weights to improve their strength. Tennis players practice their racket technique, but in addition they swim or walk to improve their endurance, lift weights to increase their muscle strength, and do a lot of stretching to help their flexibility and mobility on the court. Aerobic exercise is a requirement of any form of training.

## GETTING STARTED

When you first begin exercising, it is important not to try to do too much too quickly, especially if you have been inactive for a few months or more. You should go to your doctor for a checkup before you begin any exercise program if you are over 40 or have one or more of the following risk factors – smoke cigarettes, are obese, have high blood

## THREE WAYS TO IMPROVE YOUR FITNESS

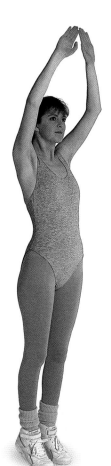

**Stretching**
*Plan a set of stretching exercises (see page 24) and do them every day. Stretching can enhance your flexibility and reduce muscle aches and pains.*

**Aerobic exercise**
*Choose a form of aerobic activity (see page 20) that you enjoy and think you would do on a regular basis. Aerobic exercises, such as brisk walking, swimming, cycling, rowing, or dancing, will improve your circulation, endurance, and the condition of your heart.*

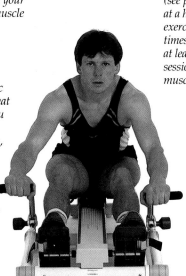

**Muscle strengthening**
*Do some muscle-strengthening exercises (see page 26) at home or at a health club. Do these exercises two to three times a week, leaving at least a day between sessions to give your muscles time to recover.*

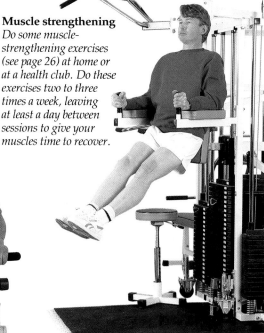

pressure, or have a family history of onset of heart disease before age 40.

If you plan to do aerobic exercise to improve the efficiency of your heart, lungs, and muscles, you need to build up to three or four sessions a week, each session lasting between 20 and 30 minutes. From that point on you may want to gradually increase the amount of time and effort you devote to exercise as your level of physical fitness improves.

## Increasing your work load

Keep a record of the time and distance you walk, run, cycle, swim, or row during each session, and build up your work load by increasing either the time or the distance by about 10 percent a week. If you feel uncomfortable at the next level, ease off a little. Remember, moderate sustained exercise will improve your cardiovascular fitness; there is no need to perform short, sharp bursts of effort.

### WALKING

Walk briskly and see how far you can go before you tire or get breathless. Your goal should be to walk 2 miles without difficulty in 30 to 45 minutes. You may need to work up to this goal gradually.

## KEEPING AN EXERCISE DIARY

Before you start your exercise program, you may want to write down what you hope to achieve. Make your goals realistic. Keeping a record of your daily exercise gives you a good overview of your efforts and will allow you to adjust your program from time to time. A week in your diary might look something like this:

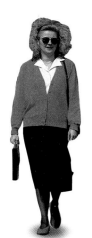

**Walking**
*Walking is an excellent form of exercise for most people.*

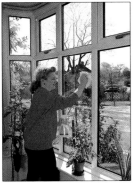

**House cleaning**
*A house-cleaning session can be a good workout if you bend and stretch with determination.*

| NAME | Carolyn Hurland |
|---|---|
| AGE | 44 |
| OCCUPATION | Newspaper editor |
| HOBBIES | Painting, bridge, some tennis |
| EXERCISE GOALS | • To increase my endurance; I often lose tennis matches because I tire after the first set<br>• To lose 5 pounds<br>• To enhance my flexibility and reduce the stiffness in my back and legs |
| DAILY EXERCISE | Daily stretching routine after dinner every evening; climb the three flights of stairs to my apartment, rather than take the elevator |
| SUNDAY | Played two sets of tennis |
| MONDAY | Walked one mile from train station to office |
| TUESDAY | Walked one mile from train station to office<br>Swam with family, evening |
| WEDNESDAY | Walked one mile from train station to office |
| THURSDAY | Walked two miles total, from train station to office and back again |
| FRIDAY | Walked one mile from train station to office |
| SATURDAY | House cleaning; walked to store |

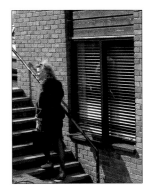

**Climbing stairs**
*Climbing a few flights of stairs every day can play a significant role in improving your fitness.*

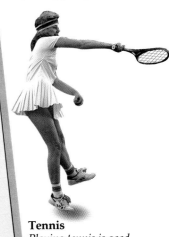

**Tennis**
*Playing tennis is good overall exercise, whether or not your backhand measures up to that of a professional athlete.*

# ARE YOU EXERCISING SAFELY?

There are many reasons for sports injuries. Some accidents are beyond your control, but many are caused by overly aggressive behavior, failure to use the correct equipment, or poor technique. It is up to you to give some thought to accident prevention.

This self-test on safety and exercise is presented in the form of a maze. Answer each question; if your answer to a question is "no," go on to the next one. If your answer is "yes," go outside the maze to the text below to learn more before you answer the next question.

## DID YOU ANSWER "YES"? THEN READ ON

**QUESTION 1**
**Action** Consult your doctor and get a checkup before you start to exercise.

**QUESTION 2**
Possible symptoms of heart trouble include chest pain or pressure; pain in the neck, jaw, or arms; palpitations; dizziness; nausea; blurred vision; light-headedness; severe breathlessness; or feeling faint.

**Action** Consult your doctor and don't exercise until your doctor says that it is safe to do so.

**QUESTION 3**
**Action** Consult your doctor for advice on appropriate exercise for you.

**QUESTION 4**
An acute infection can lead to serious complications if you do any strenuous exercise.

**Action** Rest until your infection clears up.

**QUESTION 5**
If the injury is still painful, tender, stiff, or swollen, you are not ready to return to exercising vigorously.

**Action** A little common sense should help you decide when to resume exercise. Call your doctor if you need advice.

**QUESTION 6**
Chronically stiff or sore muscles signal overtraining.

**Action** Allow yourself a little longer to recover between exercise sessions.

**QUESTION 7**
Shoes that are loose or worn down may cause injury or other problems (see page 77).

**Action** Get a new pair of shoes if yours are excessively worn, fit poorly, or are uncomfortable.

**QUESTION 8**
Protective equipment can help shield you from injury.

**Action** Find out what equipment you might need, get it, and use it.

**QUESTION 9**
Alcohol and some other drugs can cause a loss of coordination and increase your chances of injury.

**Action** Don't exercise until the effects of alcohol or the drug have worn off.

**QUESTION 10**
It is important to warm up your muscles before exercise (see page 74).

**QUESTION 11**
Some injuries are the result of using equipment that is the wrong size.

**Action** Have a professional check your equipment to be sure it is right for you.

**QUESTION 12**
Some injuries can be caused by faulty technique.

**Action** Take some lessons or read a book on technique.

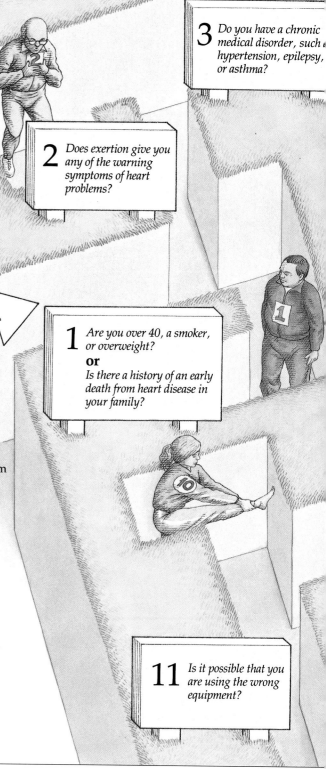

**BEGIN HERE**

**3** *Do you have a chronic medical disorder, such as hypertension, epilepsy, or asthma?*

**2** *Does exertion give you any of the warning symptoms of heart problems?*

**1** *Are you over 40, a smoker, or overweight?*
**or**
*Is there a history of an early death from heart disease in your family?*

**11** *Is it possible that you are using the wrong equipment?*

pressure, or have a family history of onset of heart disease before age 40.

If you plan to do aerobic exercise to improve the efficiency of your heart, lungs, and muscles, you need to build up to three or four sessions a week, each session lasting between 20 and 30 minutes. From that point on you may want to gradually increase the amount of time and effort you devote to exercise as your level of physical fitness improves.

## Increasing your work load

Keep a record of the time and distance you walk, run, cycle, swim, or row during each session, and build up your work load by increasing either the time or the distance by about 10 percent a week. If you feel uncomfortable at the next level, ease off a little. Remember, moderate sustained exercise will improve your cardiovascular fitness; there is no need to perform short, sharp bursts of effort.

## KEEPING AN EXERCISE DIARY

Before you start your exercise program, you may want to write down what you hope to achieve. Make your goals realistic. Keeping a record of your daily exercise gives you a good overview of your efforts and will allow you to adjust your program from time to time. A week in your diary might look something like this:

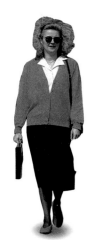

**Walking**
*Walking is an excellent form of exercise for most people.*

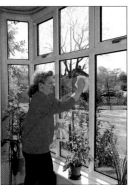

**House cleaning**
*A house-cleaning session can be a good workout if you bend and stretch with determination.*

| | |
|---|---|
| NAME | Carolyn Hurland |
| AGE | 44 |
| OCCUPATION | Newspaper editor |
| HOBBIES | Painting, bridge, some tennis |
| EXERCISE GOALS | • To increase my endurance; I often lose tennis matches because I tire after the first set<br>• To lose 5 pounds<br>• To enhance my flexibility and reduce the stiffness in my back and legs |
| DAILY EXERCISE | Daily stretching routine after dinner every evening; climb the three flights of stairs to my apartment, rather than take the elevator |
| SUNDAY | Played two sets of tennis |
| MONDAY | Walked one mile from train station to office |
| TUESDAY | Walked one mile from train station to office<br>Swam with family, evening |
| WEDNESDAY | Walked one mile from train station to office |
| THURSDAY | Walked two miles total, from train station to office and back again |
| FRIDAY | Walked one mile from train station to office |
| SATURDAY | House cleaning; walked to store |

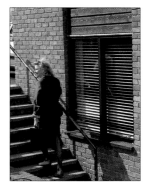

**Climbing stairs**
*Climbing a few flights of stairs every day can play a significant role in improving your fitness.*

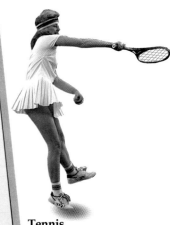

**Tennis**
*Playing tennis is good overall exercise, whether or not your backhand measures up to that of a professional athlete.*

# CHAPTER FOUR

# HOW TO EXERCISE SAFELY

## INTRODUCTION

## AVOIDING INJURY

## PREPARING YOUR BODY FOR EXERCISE

## SPORTS CLOTHING AND EQUIPMENT

## OVEREXERCISING

MOST PEOPLE ACCEPT the fact that exercise improves physical fitness and general well-being. Medical evidence provides another incentive to exercise because physical activity also protects against cardiovascular disease and some of the degenerative disorders associated with aging. As helpful as exercise is, it is important to realize that, occasionally, the result of an effort to exercise is injury, illness, and, in rare circumstances, death. Although everyone who exercises assumes some increased risk of injury, you can reduce most of the potential hazards if you pay attention to safety guidelines. In this chapter, we show you how to exercise safely while you enjoy all the benefits of exercise. The first section in this chapter, AVOIDING INJURY, discusses in detail some of the reasons exercise-induced injuries and

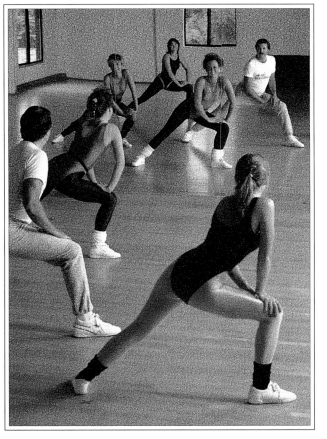

illnesses occur and some of the danger signals for those at risk of having a heart attack. Being out of shape, not recovering completely after an illness, having a faulty sports technique, or suffering from certain acute medical conditions can cause serious problems if you are not always careful. The section includes a questionnaire to help you test yourself on your exercise behavior and on your knowledge of equipment and technique. The questionnaire also can help you evaluate whether your health history suggests that you should take special precautions before you begin your exercises.

Even people who are physically fit can injure themselves if they start exercising abruptly or stop suddenly. So, even if you are in good shape, it is a good idea to warm up and cool down as part of your exercise routine. In PREPARING YOUR BODY FOR EXERCISE, we illustrate some techniques for warming up and cooling down. Another step toward reducing the risk of injury is choosing appropriate clothing and using protective equipment, especially if you are involved in competitive sports. Some guidelines are offered in SPORTS CLOTHING AND EQUIPMENT. As more and more people exercise regularly, the incidence of complications from overexercising has also increased. Problems once seen primarily in professional athletes now appear more frequently in people who exercise for their health or for recreation several times a week. Such complications range from symptoms such as muscle soreness and stiffness to injuries such as fractures. In OVEREXERCISING, we alert you to some potential dangers of exercising too much.

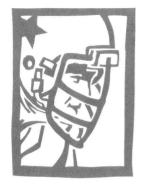

# AVOIDING INJURY

I N MOST CASES, REGULAR exercise is an excellent investment in your long-term health and physical fitness. For a few people, however, exercise can result in injury or even death. So how can you make sure you exercise safely and stay healthy?

There are several precautions that you can take to prevent an accident during your exercise or afterward.

**Exercise stress test**
*An exercise stress test assesses the way in which your heart responds to physical activity. Your pulse rate, blood pressure, and the electrical activity of your heart are recorded during a strenuous exercise, such as walking on a treadmill. If you have heart disease, the stress test may record an irregular pulse, a drop in blood pressure during exercise, or abnormal electrical impulses.*

## LACK OF FITNESS

People who are out of shape are much more likely to injure themselves when they exercise or participate in a sport than physically fit people are. Lack of fitness causes the heart to be less efficient at pumping blood to the muscles during

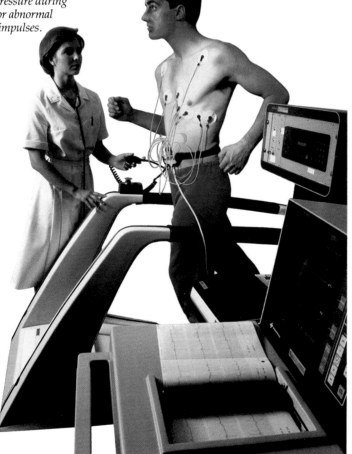

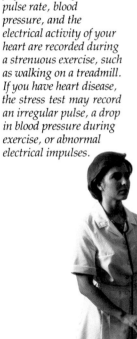

exercise. This means that your muscles are not getting enough oxygen to use as fuel for your activities. As a result, your muscles tire more rapidly, your reflexes slow down, and injury becomes more of a possibility. This is why more injuries occur toward the end of a game or a race.

Lack of physical fitness is also a common reason people are injured when they ski. They arrive on the slopes having done little or no exercise since their last skiing trip. Muscle fatigue sets in quickly, reducing coordination, and they fall and break a leg while attempting more than they are prepared for.

### Getting a checkup

If you are over 40, it is a good idea to have a checkup before embarking on an exercise program, especially if you have a family history of any chronic illness or an early death from heart disease. Although very few people die during exercise, you can place your health at serious risk if you exercise too strenuously when you have conditions such as coronary heart disease or high blood pressure.

Your doctor will perform a thorough examination, check your pulse and blood pressure, and listen to your heart and lungs. If you have high blood pressure, you may need to have it brought under control before you do any strenuous activity, and your doctor may recommend that you avoid certain exercises altogether. It is usually safe for people who have coronary heart disease to exercise (with their doctor's approval), as long as the exertion does not cause any of the warning symptoms of a heart attack (see WARNING on page 69).

## Danger signals

An important aspect of exercising safely is being able to recognize danger signals, particularly those that indicate you may be overtaxing your heart. Fainting during exercise, for example, is serious, because it implies a reduced blood flow to the brain as a result of a decrease in blood pressure or an abrupt change in the rhythm of your heart. If your heart is working properly, your blood pressure should actually increase during exercise.

Feeling faint after exercise is not normally a cause for serious concern. The sensation of feeling faint occurs in part because of a pooling of blood in your legs and can be prevented by walking, rather than standing still, after exercising.

**Skiing**
*It is important to improve your overall fitness by doing aerobic exercises and by performing strengthening exercises for your leg muscles if you are planning a skiing vacation. Skiing is a good form of exercise if you warm up first and work on your technique.*

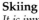

## RECENT INJURY

After any injury, make sure you have recovered completely before you resume any vigorous form of exercise that uses the injured part of your body. Otherwise, you run the risk of aggravating and prolonging the injury or even inflicting permanent damage. You are also more likely to suffer a second injury, as a result of trying to protect the painful part of your body. For example, a person with a sore foot has a tendency to run awkwardly, which can cause injury to the other foot or leg.

**Incomplete recovery**
*You can do more damage if you start to exercise before an injury (such as a sprained knee ligament) has healed.*

### WARNING

If you are exercising and become aware of any of these symptoms, stop and call for help. These symptoms may signal a heart attack:

♦ chest pain or chest pressure

♦ pain in the neck, jaw, or arms
♦ palpitations
♦ dizziness
♦ light-headedness
♦ nausea
♦ blurred vision
♦ severe breathlessness
♦ fainting or feeling faint.

## Rehabilitation

Rehabilitation after an injury usually includes exercises to restore elasticity and strength to the tissues that were injured, exercises to bring back a full range of motion, and exercises to reestablish balance and coordination. Once you can do these exercises without producing any pain, stiffness, or swelling, you are ready to start your regular exercise again. First, try to identify the cause of your injury, which may help you prevent another injury of the same type. If your injury stopped you from doing any aerobic exercises, resume them once you have recovered. Otherwise, you run the risk of being injured again.

## ALCOHOL AND OTHER DRUGS

Never drink alcohol just before exercising or even within a few hours before exercising. While a small amount of alcohol relaxes your body, it also causes a loss of coordination and a delay in your reaction time, both of which impair your performance and increase the chance of your injuring yourself.

Alcohol also increases your risk of hypothermia (a condition in which your body temperature is too low to sustain your normal bodily functions) if you are exercising in cold weather. The alcohol creates a false sense of warmth by dilating (widening) the blood vessels under your skin. This increase in blood flow may make your skin feel warm, but the alcohol actually increases the amount of heat lost from your body. Your body temperature then decreases.

### Other drugs

Like alcohol, other drugs can make you feel dizzy or drowsy and cause a sudden lapse of concentration or loss of coordination. Many drugs can have this effect, including antihistamines, diuretics, sleeping pills taken the night before exercising, and drugs of abuse.

## RUNNING

People who run or jog may experience a variety of different injuries. However, most injuries could be prevented by taking some sensible precautions.

Wear running shoes that fit well and feel comfortable (see FOOTWEAR on page 77). Replacing your running shoes promptly when they feel or look worn out will also help protect you.

Don't run on the side of a road unless you really have no other choice of a path. To avoid being hit by a car, run facing the oncoming traffic. If you run on a track, it is a good idea to vary your direction by occasionally switching between clockwise and counterclockwise circuits.

**Hazards of drugs**
*Participating in sports requires a complex synchronization of movement, good balance, and coordination. These motor skills are impaired by many drugs, including alcohol and some cold remedies.*

**Sloped roads**
*If you continually run on the same side of a highway that has a banked shoulder, you will put excessive strain on your ankles and knees, which can lead to injury. Crossing the road will ensure that the stress is distributed evenly.*

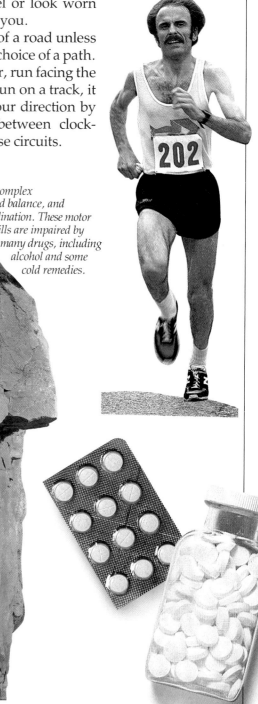

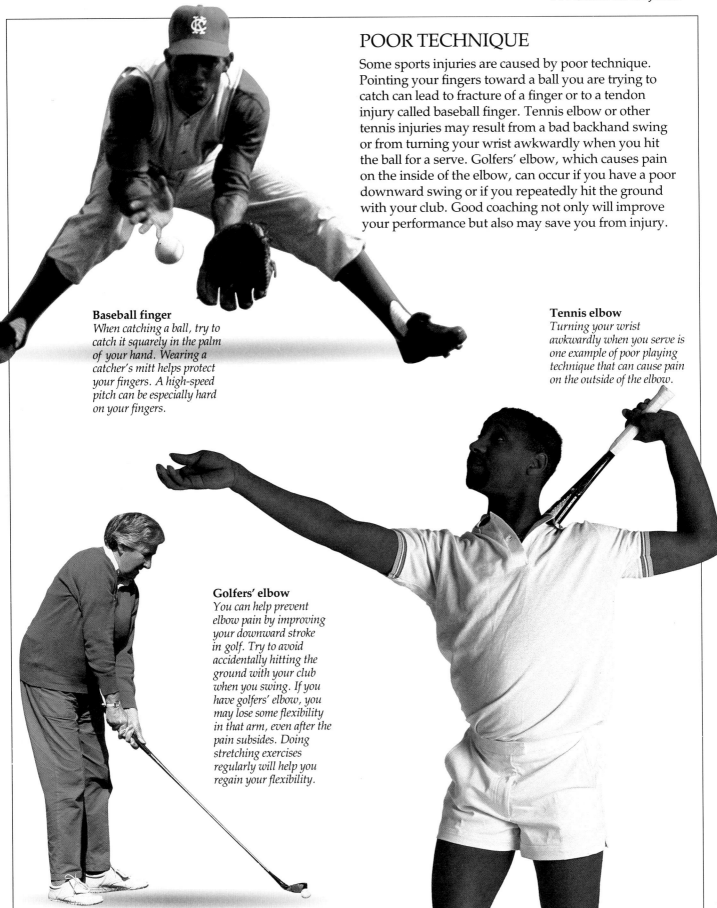

# POOR TECHNIQUE

Some sports injuries are caused by poor technique. Pointing your fingers toward a ball you are trying to catch can lead to fracture of a finger or to a tendon injury called baseball finger. Tennis elbow or other tennis injuries may result from a bad backhand swing or from turning your wrist awkwardly when you hit the ball for a serve. Golfers' elbow, which causes pain on the inside of the elbow, can occur if you have a poor downward swing or if you repeatedly hit the ground with your club. Good coaching not only will improve your performance but also may save you from injury.

**Baseball finger**
*When catching a ball, try to catch it squarely in the palm of your hand. Wearing a catcher's mitt helps protect your fingers. A high-speed pitch can be especially hard on your fingers.*

**Tennis elbow**
*Turning your wrist awkwardly when you serve is one example of poor playing technique that can cause pain on the outside of the elbow.*

**Golfers' elbow**
*You can help prevent elbow pain by improving your downward stroke in golf. Try to avoid accidentally hitting the ground with your club when you swing. If you have golfers' elbow, you may lose some flexibility in that arm, even after the pain subsides. Doing stretching exercises regularly will help you regain your flexibility.*

# ARE YOU EXERCISING SAFELY?

There are many reasons for sports injuries. Some accidents are beyond your control, but many are caused by overly aggressive behavior, failure to use the correct equipment, or poor technique. It is up to you to give some thought to accident prevention.

This self-test on safety and exercise is presented in the form of a maze. Answer each question; if your answer to a question is "no," go on to the next one. If your answer is "yes," go outside the maze to the text below to learn more before you answer the next question.

## DID YOU ANSWER "YES"?
## THEN READ ON

**QUESTION 1**
**Action** Consult your doctor and get a checkup before you start to exercise.

**QUESTION 2**
Possible symptoms of heart trouble include chest pain or pressure; pain in the neck, jaw, or arms; palpitations; dizziness; nausea; blurred vision; light-headedness; severe breathlessness; or feeling faint.

**Action** Consult your doctor and don't exercise until your doctor says that it is safe to do so.

**QUESTION 3**
**Action** Consult your doctor for advice on appropriate exercise for you.

**QUESTION 4**
An acute infection can lead to serious complications if you do any strenuous exercise.

**Action** Rest until your infection clears up.

**QUESTION 5**
If the injury is still painful, tender, stiff, or swollen, you are not ready to return to exercising vigorously.

**Action** A little common sense should help you decide when to resume exercise. Call your doctor if you need advice.

**QUESTION 6**
Chronically stiff or sore muscles signal overtraining.

**Action** Allow yourself a little longer to recover between exercise sessions.

**QUESTION 7**
Shoes that are loose or worn down may cause injury or other problems (see page 77).

**Action** Get a new pair of shoes if yours are excessively worn, fit poorly, or are uncomfortable.

**QUESTION 8**
Protective equipment can help shield you from injury.

**Action** Find out what equipment you might need, get it, and use it.

**QUESTION 9**
Alcohol and some other drugs can cause a loss of coordination and increase your chances of injury.

**Action** Don't exercise until the effects of alcohol or the drug have worn off.

**QUESTION 10**
It is important to warm up your muscles before exercise (see page 74).

**QUESTION 11**
Some injuries are the result of using equipment that is the wrong size.

**Action** Have a professional check your equipment to be sure it is right for you.

**QUESTION 12**
Some injuries can be caused by faulty technique.

**Action** Take some lessons or read a book on technique.

**3** Do you have a chronic medical disorder, such as hypertension, epilepsy, or asthma?

**2** Does exertion give you any of the warning symptoms of heart problems?

BEGIN HERE

**1** Are you over 40, a smoker, or overweight?
**or**
Is there a history of an early death from heart disease in your family?

**11** Is it possible that you are using the wrong equipment?

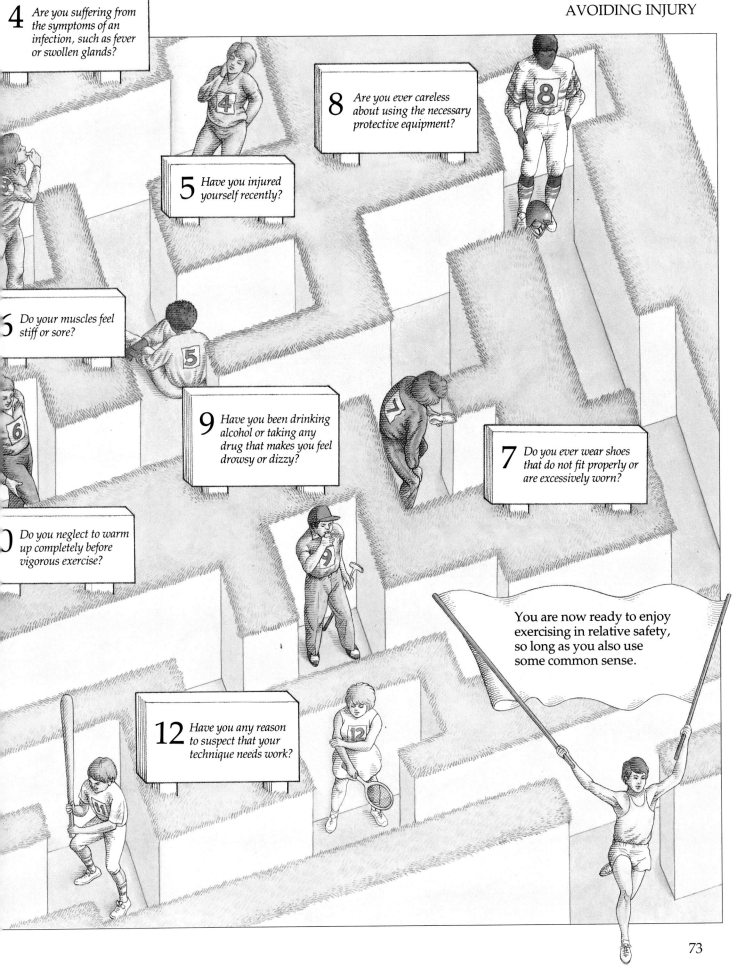

**4** Are you suffering from the symptoms of an infection, such as fever or swollen glands?

**8** Are you ever careless about using the necessary protective equipment?

**5** Have you injured yourself recently?

**6** Do your muscles feel stiff or sore?

**9** Have you been drinking alcohol or taking any drug that makes you feel drowsy or dizzy?

**7** Do you ever wear shoes that do not fit properly or are excessively worn?

Do you neglect to warm up completely before vigorous exercise?

**12** Have you any reason to suspect that your technique needs work?

You are now ready to enjoy exercising in relative safety, so long as you also use some common sense.

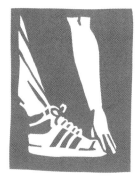

# PREPARING YOUR BODY FOR EXERCISE

HOWEVER PHYSICALLY fit you are, it is important to warm up your muscles before exercising and to cool them down afterward. Your body may "protest" with a variety of pains when you neglect to warm up. Even people who are in good condition risk injury if they suddenly start exercising strenuously without preparing their muscles for the necessary contractions or if they stop abruptly after exertion without easing their muscles back to a resting condition.

An electric motor activates your food processor or fan at the touch of a button. Your muscles do not respond so instantaneously. To meet the demands of exercise, your muscles undergo a range of physical changes; these changes should take place gradually to minimize the risk of injury. One such change in the muscles that occurs to accommodate an increased blood supply is an increase in the diameter of the blood vessels.

## WARMING UP

The best way to ensure that you warm up your muscles adequately before exercising is to establish a warm-up routine and perform it every time before you do vigorous exercise, whether you are walking for fun, training, or taking part in competition. Warming up also helps you prepare psychologically for exercise or

## HOW TO WARM UP

A complete warm-up routine should last at least 10 minutes, but don't start your warm-up too far in advance. If more than 10 minutes elapse after you finish your warm-up and before you start to exercise, your tissues will have cooled down again, and any benefit will be lost. You may want to do some brisk walking or slow jogging as your final warm-up exercise.

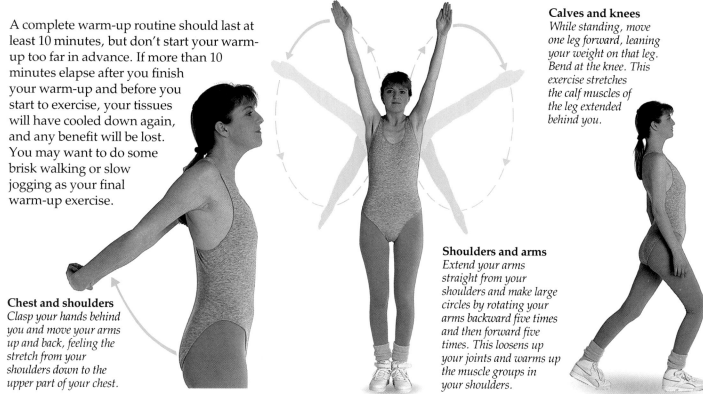

**Calves and knees**
*While standing, move one leg forward, leaning your weight on that leg. Bend at the knee. This exercise stretches the calf muscles of the leg extended behind you.*

**Chest and shoulders**
*Clasp your hands behind you and move your arms up and back, feeling the stretch from your shoulders down to the upper part of your chest.*

**Shoulders and arms**
*Extend your arms straight from your shoulders and make large circles by rotating your arms backward five times and then forward five times. This loosens up your joints and warms up the muscle groups in your shoulders.*

competition, which is an important consideration for professionals and non-professionals alike.

The main reason for warming up is to protect your muscles, tendons, and ligaments. If you start to exercise without a warm-up, you could easily tear or strain a muscle or other soft tissue while making any sudden movement that stretches it. This is especially true of activities such as throwing or kicking a ball, which requires a variety of movements by your arms and legs. Also, your body will simply feel better if you warm up your muscles before you exercise.

## Warm-up aids

Using liniment, other lotions, or creams may make you feel good, but they in no way substitute for warming up and do not help prevent muscle injury. Having a massage is also a good way to get the blood flowing through your muscles to warm them up, but the massage should be followed by a series of stretches.

## COOLING DOWN

Cooling down after exercise is important in part because it helps prevent muscle cramps from developing. To cool down, walk around for a few minutes and repeat the loosening-up exercises and muscle stretches you did in your warm-up routine. As with the warm-ups, a massage after exercise may make you feel good but is not a substitute for a cooling-down routine.

### HOW TO COOL DOWN

**Keeping mobile**
*The first principle of cooling down correctly is to taper off gradually. Never stop suddenly after an exercise. Jogging gently (below) for a few minutes after a long run, combined with a repeat of your stretching routine, ensures that the tissues of your muscle groups do not cool down too suddenly.*

**Hamstring stretch**
*Stand on one leg and pull up the other toward your chest. Gently pull the clasped leg up toward your chin. This warm-up is good for the hamstring muscles of your legs.*

**"No hands" squat**
*Lower yourself from standing upright to a squat, then stand up slowly without using your arms to help you. Repeat this exercise five times to warm up the back and thigh muscles.*

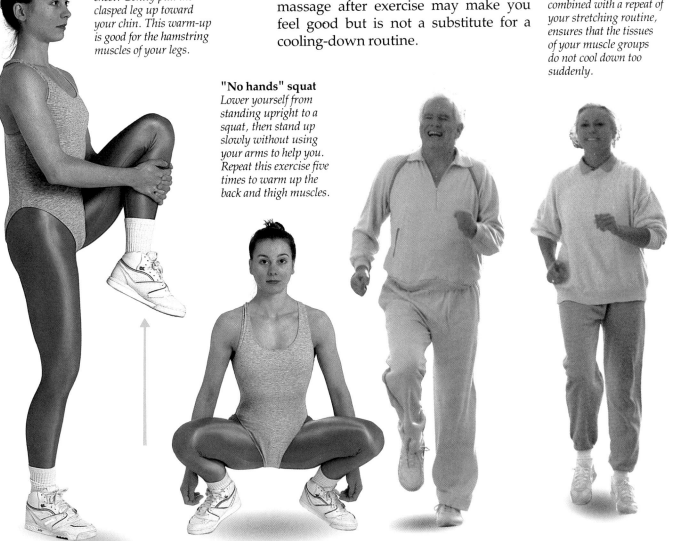

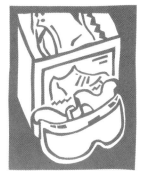

# SPORTS CLOTHING AND EQUIPMENT

APPROPRIATE CLOTHING and protective equipment are vital in helping to prevent injury during exercise. Although some injuries may be unavoidable, others are caused by inappropriate or poorly fitting clothes and by failure to use the necessary equipment. The risks involved in choosing to ride a bicycle without wearing a helmet, for example, might seem obvious; but the potential hazards of other choices, such as wearing your running shoes to play racket sports, may be less apparent.

Once you make a decision to play a sport or do some form of exercise regularly, ask an expert about the type of equipment that is most suitable for your chosen activity. (The librarian at your public library can help you find magazine articles or books about your activity if you do not choose to join a health club or gym.) Or ask a friend who has had relevant experience. It is worth investing some money in well-made equipment that offers maximum protection.

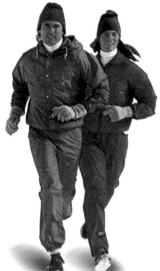

**Dressing for cold weather**
*In winter it is important to protect yourself from the cold and the wind and to keep dry. If you run in cold weather, wearing several layers of thin clothing will provide better insulation for your body than will one layer of thick material. You lose much of your body heat through your head, so wear a hat. Skiers need warm clothes, including hats.*

## JEWELRY

Always remember to remove your bracelets, watches, necklaces, or earrings before you play any contact sport. Rings should also be removed, or at least taped to help prevent finger injury.

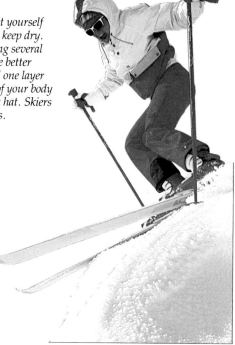

## CLOTHING

Unless you are a member of an athletic team, your choice of clothing is a matter of personal preference. However, following the guidelines below will ensure that your clothing is comfortable and offers adequate protection.

♦ Clothing should fit you neither too loosely nor too tightly.

♦ Clothes made of cotton are preferable to those made of synthetic fibers because cotton is absorbent and promotes the efficient loss of body heat by allowing the evaporation of sweat.

♦ Wear a clean set of clothes for each exercise session for good personal

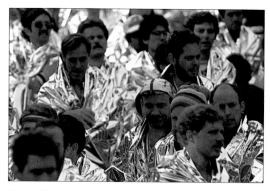

**Long-distance events**
*Lightweight shorts and shirts are comfortable and practical for running a marathon in most climates. An aluminum foil blanket is often wrapped around the runner after a race to prevent an excessive drop in body temperature.*

hygiene. Because body heat is lost as sweat evaporates, it is important in cold weather to change to dry clothing immediately after exercising if your clothing becomes drenched in perspiration.

◆ Wear comfortable underclothing made of cotton. Tight underclothing may cause chafing of the skin.

◆ Choose socks made of cotton or of a mixture of cotton and synthetic fibers, and avoid tight socks that could restrict circulation. On the other hand, blisters may form if your socks are too big and "bunch up" or rub inside your shoe.

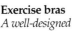

**Exercise bras**
*A well-designed sports bra should have wide shoulder straps that do not slip off the shoulder, a broad band under the bust to prevent the bra from riding up, and fasteners that do not irritate your skin.*

**Dressing for the weather**
*In hot weather, wear loose-fitting, light-colored clothing. Also, wear a hat or sun visor (below) if you are going to be in the sun. On cool days, wear a windbreaker jacket (right).*

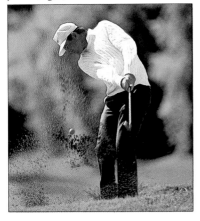

**Making yourself visible**
*If you exercise outdoors after dark, wear white or light-colored clothing and fluorescent reflecting wristbands or a headband so that drivers can see you.*

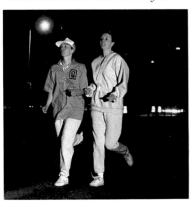

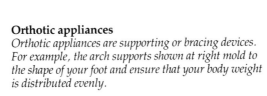

**Orthotic appliances**
*Orthotic appliances are supporting or bracing devices. For example, the arch supports shown at right mold to the shape of your foot and ensure that your body weight is distributed evenly.*

# FOOTWEAR

Shoes and boots are an important part of your protective equipment. Some exercise-induced injuries can be prevented if you replace worn-out shoes and make sure that the type of shoe you wear is suitable for your particular activity. For example, if you play golf, wear shoes with cleats to prevent slipping.

## Special footwear

Some foot problems can cause injuries such as back pain and shin splints unless you wear special footwear. Problems such as a falling arch or excessive pronation (in which the sole of the foot turns inward) can be corrected by using an orthotic appliance (a supporting or bracing device) fitted inside your shoe.

If one of your legs is significantly shorter than the other, you may need a heel elevator on your sports shoe. Continuing to play without such an aid could affect your spine and cause back pain.

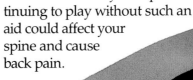

# HOW TO CHOOSE YOUR EXERCISE SHOES

Choosing shoes that are appropriate for your sport – and your feet – is vitally important. Although there are hundreds of different designs on the market, many of them are made more for fashion than they are for protecting your feet. Different activities require different shoe designs, and wearing an inappropriate shoe can result in injury. A good fit and the condition of your shoes are important, too. Wearing poorly fitting or worn-out shoes can encourage a variety of injuries, from blisters to a sprained ankle.

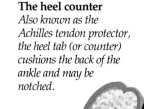

**Shoelaces**
*Tying your laces too tightly can cause inflammation of the tendons on the top of your feet. Be sure that your laces do not drag on the ground.*

## THE WELL-DESIGNED SHOE

**The heel counter**
*Also known as the Achilles tendon protector, the heel tab (or counter) cushions the back of the ankle and may be notched.*

**The tongue**
*The tongue and edging of the shoe may be padded to prevent chafing.*

**The upper part of the shoe**
*The upper part should be firm, flexible, and able to keep your foot stable. Natural materials such as leather are best.*

**Shoe width**
*If shoes are too narrow, your feet will hurt and you could be more vulnerable to injury because of the pain or because of reduced mobility. Shoes that are too tight or too loose may rub and cause blisters.*

**Cushioned insoles**
*The insole of your shoe should act as a cushion to absorb shock and reduce jarring of your heels, ankles, knees, hips, and spine. A skimpy or worn-out insole can lead to injury. The best type of insole is one that springs back to its original shape every time you take your weight off that foot. Ordinary foam usually loses its resilience quickly and will not cushion your foot each time it strikes the ground.*

**The outer sole**
*The outer sole should be able to withstand rough treatment but should not be too rigid. It should be waterproof and provide insulation from the cold.*

# WHAT SHOULD I LOOK FOR IN AN ATHLETIC SHOE?

Different exercises involve different types of movement. Activities that require movement in different directions – for example, aerobic dancing – require shoes with a strong pad under the ball of the foot and material with a little "give" around the heel to make sure that the heel is not held rigid. Running shoes would not be suitable for aerobic dancing because they have a rigid heel support and a flexible front, which allows the foot to bend, but does not provide the necessary protection to the ball of the foot.

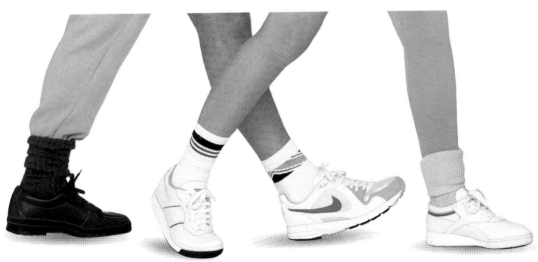

**Walking shoes**
*Walking shoes should have a sturdy sole to accommodate walking on pavement and other rough surfaces. The soles should also provide support for your arches.*

**Tennis shoes**
*The foot moves in all directions during tennis, so shoes are designed for maximum grip on the playing surface. The upper shoe is cushioned for protection.*

**Running shoes**
*Some styles of running shoes have been designed to provide a special elevated heel that absorbs some of the impact of the foot when it hits the ground.*

**Aerobic shoes**
*Aerobic shoes should be lightweight and have a flexible sole. Shoes of this type are ideal for dancing or jogging in place but do not provide enough support for running.*

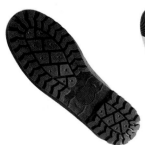

**Thick soles with grooves for extra cushioning on pavement and roads**

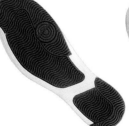

**Flexible rubber soles with narrow grooves and a pivot under the ball of the foot**

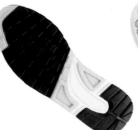

**Thick, grooved soles to withstand the impact of running on uneven surfaces**

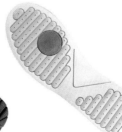

**Light, flexible soles designed for use on polished wooden dance floors**

| Pavement | Indoor composition court | Gravel | Wood |

**Ground surfaces**
*The soles of your athletic shoes may be grooved to help you get better traction. Some soles are more durable than others for particular ground surfaces; aerobic shoes won't last long if you use them on gravel.*

# PROTECTIVE EQUIPMENT

Today's consumer can choose from an enormous variety of equipment designed to protect the body from the impact of possible collisions with moving objects (such as a ball, hockey puck, or lacrosse stick), with the ground, or with other players. Manufacturers are researching ways to increase the effectiveness of protective equipment regularly, so it is worthwhile for you to periodically check the new designs.

## For your head and face

Medical experts recommend protective headgear when you are participating in any sport that carries a risk of receiving a heavy blow to the head, such as ice hockey, football, cycling, or horseback riding. Helmets are especially important for children, whether they are playing on a football team or simply riding their bicycles. Parents who enjoy taking their toddlers for a bike ride can choose from a wide variety of headgear designed for youngsters.

A mouth guard is recommended when playing most contact sports to protect your teeth, lips, tongue, inside of your mouth, and dental work. Also, a mouth guard reduces the risk of a concussion or a fractured jaw.

Never underestimate the risk of eye injury. Several squash players have suffered blindness as a result of being hit in the eye with a fast ball. Racquetball and handball players are at equal risk. If you play any of these sports, always wear goggles when you are on the court.

## For your body

Wearing well-designed protective clothing is absolutely essential for certain sports. For example, ice hockey, baseball, football, and fencing would be extremely dangerous without specialized face masks or helmets, shields, pads, and gloves.

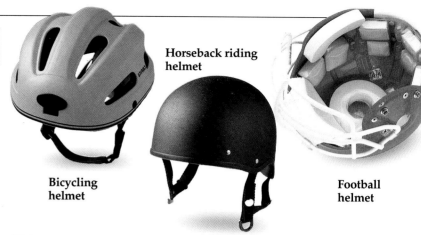

**Horseback riding helmet**

**Bicycling helmet**

**Football helmet**

**Helmets**
*Most helmets have a fiberglass or plastic outer shell and an inner lining of resilient material to absorb single violent blows or multiple softer blows. Carefully examine any helmet you plan to buy and try to determine from the labeling or packaging if the product has been tested or endorsed by any nationally known organization. Any helmet that has been dropped or subjected to a heavy blow should be checked by a professional to determine if it is still intact or requires replacing.*

**Using a mouth guard**
*Ideally, a mouth guard should be made to measure by a dentist so that it fits well and cannot be displaced easily. A mouth guard is of no use if you have to hold it in position by clenching your teeth or if it makes it difficult for you to speak or breathe through your mouth. If wearing your mouth guard causes you to feel nauseated, it probably extends too far back in your mouth.*

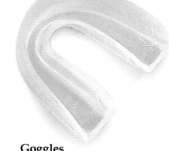

**Goggles**
*Goggles made of shatterproof plastic can significantly reduce the risk of eye injury in sports such as handball and racquetball. They also minimize irritation from chlorine in swimming pools. If you wear corrective lenses and find it uncomfortable to wear goggles over your glasses, you may want to invest in goggles with prescription lenses.*

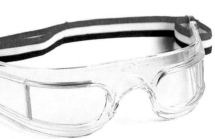

**Racquetball goggles**

**Skiing goggles**

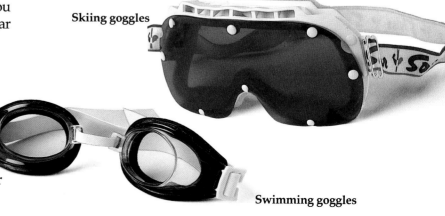

**Swimming goggles**

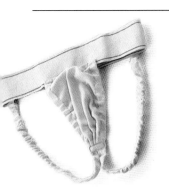

**Athletic supporter**
*Men who play sports in which extensive protection is not required (such as basketball) often wear an athletic supporter, or jockstrap, to protect their genitals.*

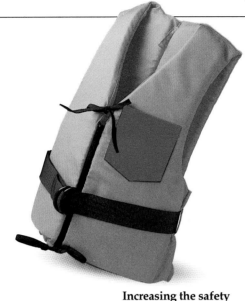

**Increasing the safety of water sports**
*Water sports are potentially dangerous because a fall or blow to the head may render you unconscious and susceptible to drowning. Even competent swimmers should wear a life jacket like the one shown above for sports such as boating, waterskiing, and canoeing.*

## TAPING

Supporting a joint with a firmly wrapped elastic bandage or adhesive tape is called taping or strapping. Doctors often recommend taping following recovery from a ligament injury to help strengthen the joint and reduce the risk of an additional injury. However, taping is never recommended to compensate for an incomplete recovery from an injury.

Taping is used preventively in collegiate or professional sports such as football and basketball to reduce the risk of joint injuries from excessive twisting during play. Trainers often use preventive taping on professional athletes who have sustained knee, leg, or ankle injuries – long after the injury has healed.

**Taping**
*An adhesive tape may be wound around the knee, ankle, or wrist to provide support. Taping that has been applied incorrectly could be a hazard in itself, so you should not attempt taping unless you have received instruction from an expert such as a doctor, nurse, or coach.*

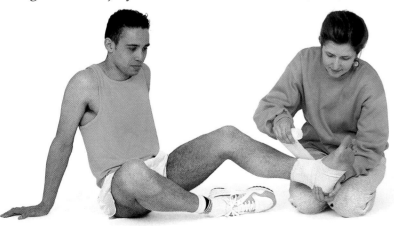

# ASK YOUR DOCTOR
## SPORTS CLOTHING AND EQUIPMENT

**Q** **My parents want me to wear my older brother's football helmet and shoulder pads when I try out for my high school team; the helmet fits fine but the shoulder pads are too big. Is it safe to wear protective equipment that is too big or too small?**

**A** No. Shoulder pads that are too big will "give" and move too much during a block or tackle. Equipment that is too small could actually cause an injury. Ask your coach if you can borrow shoulder pads that fit for the tryouts; buy new ones that fit if you play regularly.

**Q** **I have just finished a course of physical therapy after a knee operation and have been advised to tape my knee before I exercise. How should I apply this tape?**

**A** Ask a doctor or other knowledgeable person to show you the correct taping technique. It is dangerous to apply tape too tightly, and useless if it is too loose. You may find that an elastic bandage, which is easier to put on, will support your knee adequately.

**Q** **All the experienced players at my racquetball club wear goggles when they play. I'm just a beginner and hate the way goggles feel. Do I need them?**

**A** Yes. Any person – novice or expert – who plays racquetball or handball needs eye protection. If you find your goggles very uncomfortable, invest in a more expensive, better-designed pair. Eventually, putting on your goggles will become as much a part of dressing for your game as putting on your shoes.

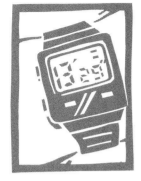

# OVEREXERCISING

T O AVOID OVEREXERCISING, always allow yourself enough time to recover adequately from your last exercise session. Do not attempt any strenuous physical activity if you have any muscle soreness or stiffness as a result of your last workout. Even mild pain may interfere with your coordination and render you liable to an injury.

Three or four sessions of moderate physical activity a week, each lasting at least 30 minutes, are enough to keep most people fit. There is no need to "go for the burn" to be healthy. For most people, it is ideal to participate in some form of gentle, regular activity such as walking five days a week. A more strenuous exercise routine, such as a heavy workout in a gym or swimming 50 lengths of a pool, should normally be undertaken only on alternate days – even by athletes in good condition. Your muscles need a day to recover between consecutive sessions.

## MUSCLE RECOVERY

The usual recovery time for muscles that have been worked to their maximum capacity is about 48 hours. During this time they may feel a little stiff and sore. These symptoms may be caused by minor damage to individual muscle fibers. You are most apt to feel stiff if you have just recently started on an exercise program.

Muscle discomfort and stiffness normally ease within the first 2 days after exertion as the muscle fibers heal. You may, however, actually feel more sore on the second day of your recovery.

**When you push yourself too hard**
*Occasionally people become almost obsessed with their exercise programs and begin pushing themselves too hard. They may become sick, injured, or exhausted and perform well below their usual standards.*

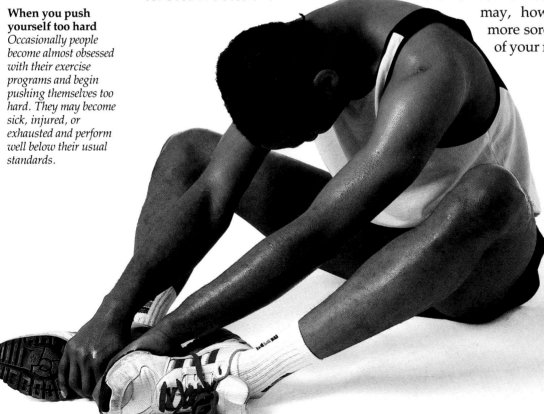

### OVERDOING IT

Symptoms that suggest that your exercise program is too demanding include
◆ muscle stiffness or soreness that has persisted since your last exercise session
◆ loss of enthusiasm
◆ reduced appetite
◆ waking up feeling tired or listless
◆ sudden unplanned loss of weight.

# DISORDERS CAUSED BY EXERCISE

Sore muscles are not the only symptom that can develop if you exercise too hard; there are also a number of specific disorders that are caused, as a whole or in part, by doing too much vigorous exercise.

### Runners' hematuria

Running a long-distance event can occasionally cause hematuria (blood in the urine). The exact cause of this is unknown, but hematuria does not necessarily signal a disease. Usually the urine is free of blood within 2 days; however, you should see a doctor promptly if the discolored urine is accompanied by difficulty in urinating, discomfort while urinating, decreased urine output, or pain in your side.

### Heat exhaustion

Strenuous exercise in hot weather can lead to heat exhaustion, in which you experience dizziness, nausea, fatigue, and sometimes cramps in your arms, legs, back, and abdomen. Heat exhaustion is caused by a failure of the body's sensitive heat-regulating mechanism (controlled by the brain) and, if untreated, can lead to a life-threatening heat stroke.

To prevent heat exhaustion, drink plenty of water before exercising in hot, humid weather, and wear lightweight, loose-fitting clothing. If you are not accustomed to exercising outdoors in hot conditions, build up gradually the amount of time you put in. If you feel any of the above symptoms while exercising outdoors in hot weather, stop immediately, rest in the shade, drink some cool water if it is available, and consult a doctor.

### Runners' diarrhea

Loose bowel movements, sometimes with visible blood and

**Inflammation of the bowel**
*The symptoms of runners' diarrhea usually disappear as soon as the person eases up substantially on his or her running schedule.*

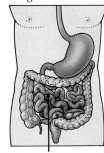

**Blood is diverted from the bowel**

**Pituitary gland**

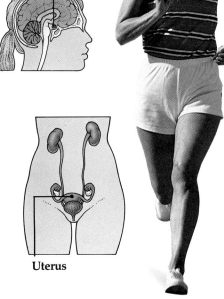

**Uterus**

mucus, may occur if you train excessively for long-distance running. It is thought to be due to ischemic colitis (inflammation of the bowel lining), which occurs as a result of a prolonged reduction in the flow of oxygen-carrying blood to the bowel lining.

During exercise, blood is usually diverted away from all parts of the digestive tract, including the bowel, to enable a larger volume of blood to service the muscles.

### Amenorrhea

Many women who exercise hard find that their periods become light and irregular. Amenorrhea (a condition in which menstruation stops altogether) sometimes develops. The cause of amenorrhea may be an exercise-induced reduction in the level of certain hormones (follicle-stimulating hormone and luteinizing hormone) produced by the pituitary gland at the base of the brain; these hormones help control the menstrual cycle. An absence of menstrual periods may also occur if a woman's weight drops substantially below the normal body weight for her height and age. You should consult a doctor if your menstrual periods stop. Generally, however, as soon as a woman cuts back on her exercise schedule, a normal menstrual cycle returns within a few months. There is usually no long-term loss of fertility.

**Menstrual changes**
*Because regular, strenuous exercise is only one possible cause of irregular menstruation or absence of menstrual periods, always discuss this symptom with your doctor.*

# CHAPTER FIVE

# SPORTS INJURIES AROUND THE BODY

## INTRODUCTION

## COMMON SITES OF INJURIES

## INJURIES TO THE HEAD AND TORSO

## INJURIES TO THE UPPER LIMBS

## INJURIES TO THE LOWER LIMBS

THE MANY BENEFITS of exercise and sports are balanced by some risks of injury. On occasion, even those who are in good condition and who exercise regularly may have an injury. The increasing availability of opportunities to exercise and play sports today has brought with it a corresponding increase in the number of sports-related injuries. In fact, most sports injuries are minor sprains, strains, or contusions (bruises) that probably do not need care from a doctor. Some injuries are more serious, of course, and require the immediate attention of a doctor. Very few injuries require hospitalization, especially injuries in those who exercise regularly to keep in shape. It is rare for a sports injury to cause irreversible damage, but a small minority of participants, particularly those taking part in hazardous contact sports, sometimes end up with a permanent disability. The good news is that most sports injuries can be avoided and that, even if you are injured, you can prevent the injury from getting worse and speed your own recovery.

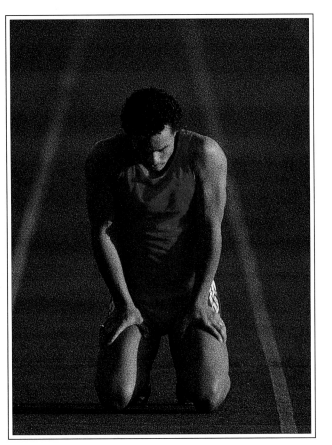

In this chapter we describe the types of injuries that may occur in sporting activities, first giving a general view and then addressing in detail INJURIES TO THE HEAD AND TORSO. Head injuries occur most often in sports that involve powerful body contact, in sports where falls occur, and in sports that carry a risk of being struck by a ball. We discuss concussion and what to do when someone loses consciousness after a head injury. A review of injuries to the neck, back, chest, and abdomen follows, including advice such as how to handle a possible neck injury on a playing field. The next section, INJURIES TO THE UPPER LIMBS, examines injuries to the shoulder, upper arm, elbow, forearm, wrist, hand, and fingers. This is followed by INJURIES TO THE LOWER LIMBS, which describes some sports injuries that affect the foot, ankle, lower leg, knee, thigh, hip, and groin.

This chapter does not attempt to teach you how to diagnose your own injury, because different types of injury produce similar symptoms. Accurate diagnosis is the job of a doctor, orthopedic surgeon, or sports medicine specialist who is experienced in the treatment of injuries. A doctor makes a diagnosis by taking into consideration your description of your symptoms, the circumstances of the injury, and the results of a physical examination; occasionally, some type of imaging is needed to confirm a diagnosis.

# COMMON SITES OF INJURIES

ANY PART OF THE BODY may be injured during sports or exercises, but some injuries occur more frequently than others. Some of the most common are joint and ligament sprains (see SPRAIN VERSUS STRAIN on page 92). If a sport or physical activity requires that you repeat a movement over and over, the part of the body used to make that movement may be prone to injury.

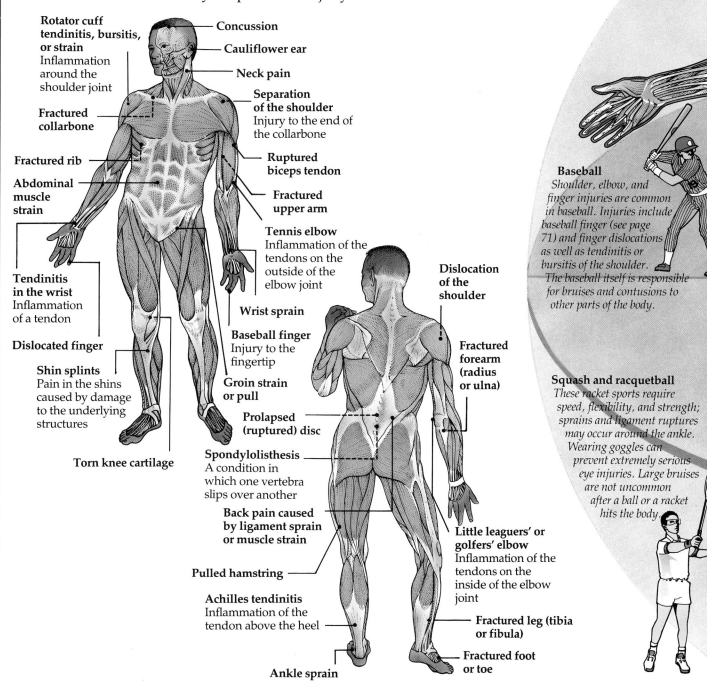

**Rotator cuff tendinitis, bursitis, or strain**
Inflammation around the shoulder joint

**Fractured collarbone**

**Fractured rib**

**Abdominal muscle strain**

**Tendinitis in the wrist**
Inflammation of a tendon

**Dislocated finger**

**Shin splints**
Pain in the shins caused by damage to the underlying structures

**Torn knee cartilage**

**Concussion**

**Cauliflower ear**

**Neck pain**

**Separation of the shoulder**
Injury to the end of the collarbone

**Ruptured biceps tendon**

**Fractured upper arm**

**Tennis elbow**
Inflammation of the tendons on the outside of the elbow joint

**Wrist sprain**

**Baseball finger**
Injury to the fingertip

**Groin strain or pull**

**Prolapsed (ruptured) disc**

**Spondylolisthesis**
A condition in which one vertebra slips over another

**Back pain caused by ligament sprain or muscle strain**

**Pulled hamstring**

**Achilles tendinitis**
Inflammation of the tendon above the heel

**Ankle sprain**

**Dislocation of the shoulder**

**Fractured forearm (radius or ulna)**

**Little leaguers' or golfers' elbow**
Inflammation of the tendons on the inside of the elbow joint

**Fractured leg (tibia or fibula)**

**Fractured foot or toe**

**Baseball**
*Shoulder, elbow, and finger injuries are common in baseball. Injuries include baseball finger (see page 71) and finger dislocations as well as tendinitis or bursitis of the shoulder. The baseball itself is responsible for bruises and contusions to other parts of the body.*

**Squash and racquetball**
*These racket sports require speed, flexibility, and strength; sprains and ligament ruptures may occur around the ankle. Wearing goggles can prevent extremely serious eye injuries. Large bruises are not uncommon after a ball or a racket hits the body.*

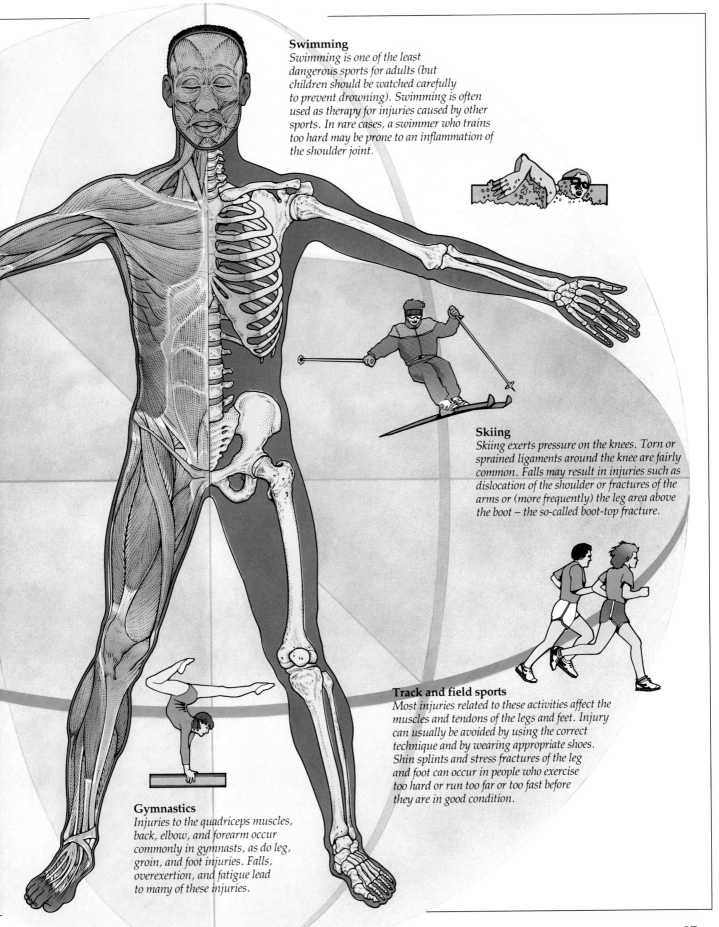

**Swimming**

*Swimming is one of the least dangerous sports for adults (but children should be watched carefully to prevent drowning). Swimming is often used as therapy for injuries caused by other sports. In rare cases, a swimmer who trains too hard may be prone to an inflammation of the shoulder joint.*

**Skiing**

*Skiing exerts pressure on the knees. Torn or sprained ligaments around the knee are fairly common. Falls may result in injuries such as dislocation of the shoulder or fractures of the arms or (more frequently) the leg area above the boot – the so-called boot-top fracture.*

**Track and field sports**

*Most injuries related to these activities affect the muscles and tendons of the legs and feet. Injury can usually be avoided by using the correct technique and by wearing appropriate shoes. Shin splints and stress fractures of the leg and foot can occur in people who exercise too hard or run too far or too fast before they are in good condition.*

**Gymnastics**

*Injuries to the quadriceps muscles, back, elbow, and forearm occur commonly in gymnasts, as do leg, groin, and foot injuries. Falls, overexertion, and fatigue lead to many of these injuries.*

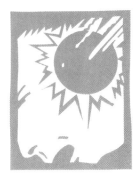

# INJURIES TO THE HEAD AND TORSO

THE SKULL, SPINE, RIB CAGE, and abdominal muscles protect the organs in the head, chest, and abdomen. These organs – including the brain, heart, lungs, and abdominal organs – are infrequently damaged during sports; much more common are injuries to the muscles, tendons, ligaments, and other soft tissues that cover and support the bones of the torso and head.

## HEAD INJURIES

Head injuries occur most often in sports that involve body contact or the risk of falling or being struck by a ball. A blow to the head may affect the brain and cause a concussion, sometimes accompanied by a temporary loss of consciousness. A concussion is caused by a disruption of nerve activity in the brain. Symptoms such as headache, nausea, dizziness, unsteadiness, blurred vision, loss of memory, and impaired concentration are

## TYPES OF HEAD INJURIES

**Infection**
In rare cases, there is a risk of infection if the skull is pierced and any foreign matter enters. Untreated, such infections may be fatal.

**Concussion**
Injuries to the head may cause a concussion – a sudden jarring of the brain, sometimes with loss of consciousness.

**Swelling**
Severe head injuries may cause swelling that can damage the brain, since it is enclosed in the skull and therefore has no room to expand.

**Brain damage**
Head injuries may lead to permanent damage or death of nerve cells, resulting in impaired brain function. Brain damage may also be the end result of repeated concussions.

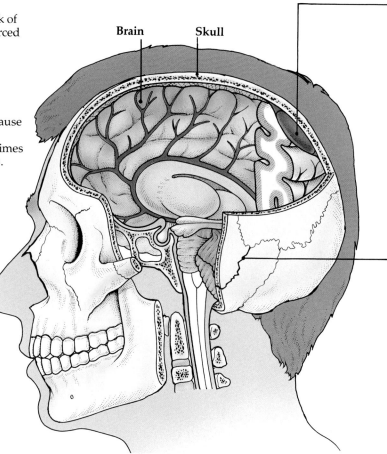

Brain  Skull

**Hemorrhage and hematoma**
A head injury can cause bleeding inside or around the brain (hemorrhage). In either case, a pool of blood may collect and a blood clot may form (hematoma). If not diagnosed promptly, hematoma may lead to permanent brain damage and disability or death.

**Fracture**
A skull fracture may be confined to the skull (closed fracture), or the bone may break through the skin (open fracture). Most fractures do not affect the brain. In rare cases, fragments of the skull may be driven into the brain, leading to infection or brain hemorrhage, which can be fatal.

# FIRST AID FOR LOSS OF CONSCIOUSNESS

If someone remains unconscious after a head injury, it is essential to make sure that he or she is breathing and has a heartbeat. Do not move the victim if there is a possibility of a neck or back injury. Get someone to call an ambulance and make sure that the unconscious person is not left alone.

**1** Check inside the victim's mouth to make sure that the airway is not obstructed. Remove any mouth guard, dentures, loose teeth, or dirt and make sure that the tongue has not fallen to the back of the throat. To keep the victim's airway open, tilt the head back by placing one hand on the victim's forehead and then placing the fingers of your other hand under the bones of the chin. If you are worried that the victim's neck may be broken, move only the jaw.

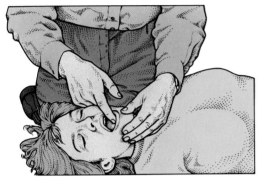

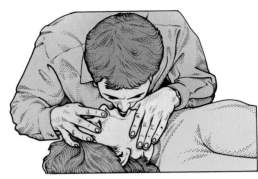

**2** If necessary, and if you have been trained in the technique, restore breathing by artificial resuscitation. If your attempt to restart breathing fails and you cannot detect a pulse in the neck, start cardiopulmonary resuscitation (CPR). Give CPR only if you have been thoroughly trained in the correct technique and you are certain that the heart has stopped beating.

**3** If there is no evidence of neck or back injury and breathing is normal, turn the victim's head to the side to prevent him or her from inhaling vomit. This is important because many people vomit as they regain consciousness. If the victim is pale and clammy, or has a rapid pulse, he or she may be in shock. Loosen any tight clothing and wrap the victim in a coat or blanket.

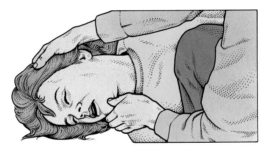

likely to develop in anyone who has a concussion. These symptoms may last from a few hours to a few days. The longer you are unconscious, the more serious the damage to your brain may be, and the more severe and prolonged your symptoms may be. In rare cases, a head injury damages the brain without causing any loss of consciousness.

## What action should you take?

If you or a friend lose consciousness after a blow to the head, even for several seconds, stop exercising and call a doctor immediately. People who continue to play after being knocked out risk aggravating the concussion or damaging the brain or its coverings further.

Even if you do not lose consciousness, consult a doctor after a blow to the head if you feel faint, dizzy, confused, nauseated, or disoriented or if you experience visual problems. Your doctor may recommend an X-ray to make sure that you have not fractured your skull, or he or she may want you to go to the hospital for observation. These precautions help diagnose the small number of cases in which a brain hemorrhage develops after an injury.

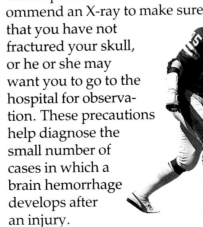

Wearing a helmet may be the single most important step you can take to prevent bicycling- or motorcycling-related injury. Head injuries account for between 50 and 75 percent of all the hospitalizations and fatalities caused by cycling, yet the risk of head injury is reduced by more than 75 percent simply by wearing a helmet. Buy and use a helmet that fits well and features a shock-absorbing lining. Wear it every time you use your bicycle, even on very short trips; many accidents occur close to home. This is especially important for children who are both riders and passengers.

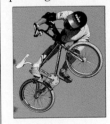

# INJURIES TO THE NECK AND BACK

An injury to the neck or back usually is in the form of a sprain or strain of the spinal ligaments, discs, or muscles, or inflammation of the muscle attachments. Any movement of your back may aggravate the pain that usually follows these injuries, and you may need to limit your physical activities for a time. Occasionally a process (prominent extension) of a vertebra in your back may be broken. Very violent accidents may cause enough damage to the vertebrae to injure the spinal cord also.

Your spine consists of a column of 24 linked vertebrae that are held in position by a complex web of ligaments and muscles.

### Injuries to the mid (thoracic) spine

Injuries to the middle part of your back are usually caused by twisting awkwardly, especially if you are carrying, lifting, pulling, or throwing a weight at the same time (as you do when you throw a discus). You can also injure this area by repeating a twisting movement, such as a tennis or golf shot, or by overreaching on each stroke in rowing. The injury is usually a strain of a muscle or ligament that causes spasms in the muscles of the middle part of your back. The pain and tenderness may spread around the side of your chest because of pressure on one of the spinal nerves that emerges from between the vertebrae.

### Injuries to the lower (lumbar-sacral) spine

Injuries to the lower part of your spine can occur when you lift a heavy weight, especially if you lift it awkwardly or twist into a position that stretches the supporting ligaments and muscles. Injuries can also result from repeated back movements that require powerful contractions, such as those you use in rowing, gymnastics, football, or playing golf. Many spinal injuries associated with exercise result from using an incorrect technique.

## TYPES OF BACK INJURIES

### Injuries to the cervical spine

You can strain the neck muscles that adjoin the cervical spine while playing any sport that involves repeated twisting of your head, such as throwing a baseball to first base. The pain is usually felt on one side of the neck only, making certain head and shoulder movements painful. The pain may also travel to your shoulder and down your arm.

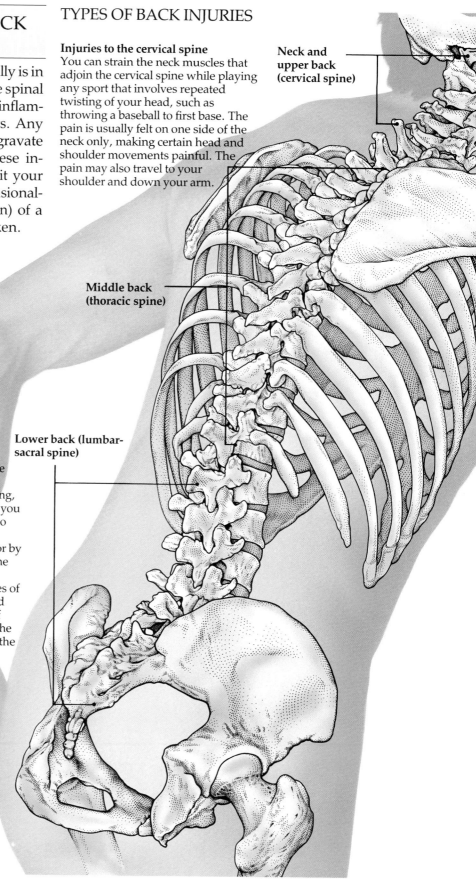

**Neck and upper back (cervical spine)**

**Middle back (thoracic spine)**

**Lower back (lumbar-sacral spine)**

The vertebrae are separated by discs of dense connective tissue, the centers of which are filled with a gelatinous substance. Each disc absorbs the stress that occurs when you move your body.

## Cervical strain (whiplash)

The sudden forward-and-backward snapping motion of the neck that occurs in an automobile accident or a violent head-on tackle can cause pain and stiffness in the neck that may feel worse a day or more after the injury if the muscles in your neck go into spasm. Cervical strain, or whiplash, is difficult to diagnose. If the injury is severe there is a risk that one or more vertebrae in the neck may be broken or dislocated. The neck should be immobilized immediately after the injury with a foam collar or a folded newspaper held in place by a scarf or towel. The person should be lifted on a board or stretcher, to prevent the head from moving independently of the body, and taken for X-ray examination.

## Prolapsed disc

A very common condition that occurs in sports or other daily activities is a prolapsed, or ruptured, intervertebral disc (also called a "slipped" disc). The lumbar discs near the base of the spine account for a large proportion of the prolapsed discs that occur.

A sudden motion, such as leaning over to pick up a weight, can rupture the disc. Actually, the disc does not shatter, but a break in the outer layer allows its soft center to protrude. The disc then presses on the nerves associated with the spinal cord, causing severe pain. (See also the CASE HISTORY on page 133.)

## CERVICAL STRAIN INJURIES

Strain of the neck can occur when a blow to the head or body causes your neck to snap rapidly and forcibly backward (below left), then forward (below right). Sudden twisting or stretching of the neck can cause several types of injury, including strain of the neck ligaments and muscles or disc rupture. All these injuries can also occur in other parts of the spine as a result of too much straining, a fall, or many other types of accidents.

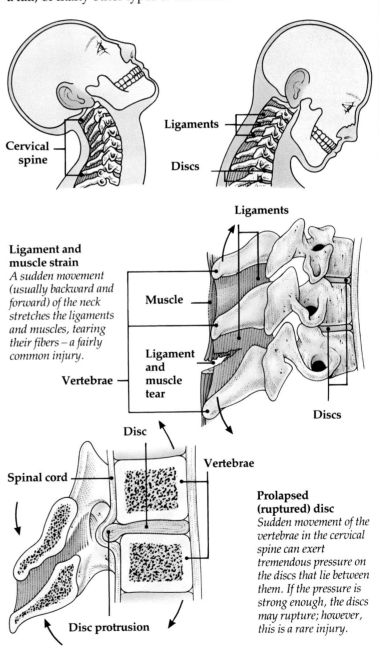

Cervical spine

Ligaments

Discs

Ligaments

**Ligament and muscle strain**
*A sudden movement (usually backward and forward) of the neck stretches the ligaments and muscles, tearing their fibers – a fairly common injury.*

Muscle

Vertebrae

Ligament and muscle tear

Discs

Disc

Vertebrae

Spinal cord

**Prolapsed (ruptured) disc**
*Sudden movement of the vertebrae in the cervical spine can exert tremendous pressure on the discs that lie between them. If the pressure is strong enough, the discs may rupture; however, this is a rare injury.*

Disc protrusion

# INJURIES TO THE ABDOMEN

The abdominal muscles and ribs protect the vital internal organs – including the stomach, liver, and spleen – and help support the spine. Weakness of the abdominal muscles may encourage poor posture and can sometimes cause back pain.

## Damage to the muscles

It is possible to tear an abdominal muscle if you receive a direct blow to your abdomen just when the muscle contracts, as sometimes happens during wrestling or boxing or when a hockey player is hit in the abdomen with a stick or puck. An abdominal muscle tear can also be caused by overstretching, which may occur during sports such as pole-vaulting or weight lifting.

A strain or tear causes pain and tenderness in the damaged area of the abdominal muscle and is usually aggravated by any movement of the trunk. To speed your recovery, you can begin gentle stretching exercises once the pain eases, usually within 2 days.

## A blow to the abdomen

A blow to the abdomen may cause you to collapse and crumple to the floor or

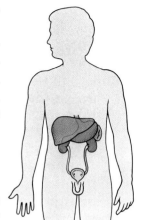

## TYPES OF ABDOMINAL INJURIES

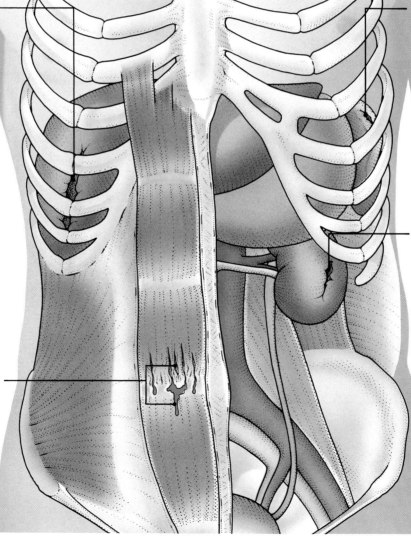

**Rupture of the liver**
The liver can rupture as a result of a hard blow to the upper right-hand part of the abdomen below the rib cage. Rupture of the liver causes bile and blood to flow into the abdominal cavity and can result in peritonitis (inflammation of the lining of the abdominal cavity), which may be fatal.

**Muscle strain and tear**
Straining and tearing your muscles, which can be caused by overstretching or by getting hit by a ball or a person, causes pain and tenderness in the damaged area. Swelling may be caused by a hematoma (a blood clot).

**Rupture of the spleen**
A rupture of the spleen and its surrounding capsule causes severe bleeding into the abdominal cavity and may be fatal. A ruptured spleen may be caused by a direct blow to the upper left-hand part of the abdomen.

**Rupture of a kidney**
A direct blow to the kidney area can cause a kidney to tear or rupture, which in turn causes blood to appear in the urine.

**Losing your breath**
A blow to the abdomen may leave you lying doubled up on the ground for a brief period. This happens because a direct blow overstimulates the bundle of nerves (solar plexus) that lies behind the breastbone.

ground, and your skin may become pale and clammy. The blow may also briefly make you feel faint or feel nauseated, and it may cause you difficulty in getting your breath. Having the breath knocked out of you is caused by a blow to the solar plexus – the bundle of nerves that lies behind the lower end of your breastbone. Your symptoms usually improve with rest within a few minutes. It is advisable to lie down or to bend forward briefly until you get your breath back.

## Internal damage

In rare cases, a severe blow to the abdomen may cause damage to an internal organ or may rupture a blood vessel in the muscle wall. If you feel sick for more than about 30 minutes after any such blow, consult your doctor at once.

A hard blow to the upper left-hand side of the abdomen may cause another rare injury, damage to your spleen, which results in immediate internal bleeding, severe abdominal pain, and shock. This type of injury causes sweating and a cold, clammy skin and may result in collapse. An emergency operation may be necessary to control the bleeding and to remove the spleen. A delayed rupture may also occur several days after the injury, at which time surgery may be required promptly.

**A torn muscle**
*Overstretching a muscle can cause it to tear. A torn muscle may be painful for several days and requires rest.*

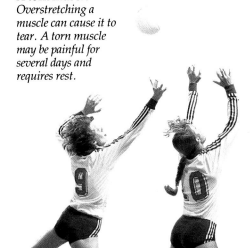

## WHAT IS A STITCH?

A sharp pain that begins suddenly in your side during strenuous exercise is commonly called a stitch. The exact cause of a stitch is unknown, but in some cases it may be the result of a spasm of the diaphragm muscle. A stitch is more likely to occur if you exercise within an hour after eating, and it is more common in people who are out of shape. It also occurs in people who are very tense.

### Easing the pain
Pain from a stitch in the side usually subsides rapidly as soon as you rest. Sometimes you can ease the pain while continuing to exercise by taking a few deep breaths and bending forward or leaning away from the side that hurts. Of course, you should stop exercising immediately if the pain gets worse or if you have reason to think the pain could have a more serious cause.

**Internal damage**
*A rider who is thrown and kicked by a horse or steer – for example, during a rodeo event (below) – may suffer serious damage to an internal organ or rupture of a blood vessel inside the muscle wall.*

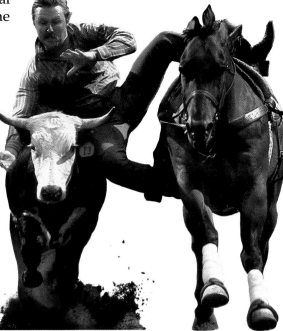

### WARNING

Abdominal pain that starts during or after exercise may or may not be caused by muscle strain or another minor injury. The pain could also be caused by lung or heart disease or by any disease involving one of the internal abdominal organs. These diseases or disorders include appendicitis, gallstones, peptic ulcers, and gynecological problems. If an abdominal pain after exercise persists for longer than 4 hours, consult your doctor promptly.

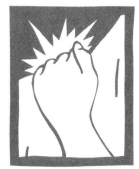

# INJURIES TO THE UPPER LIMBS

THE ARM CONTAINS 72 MUSCLES, a fact that accounts for its wide range of complex movements. Injuries to the arm muscles are more common in sports where a bat or racket is used (particularly baseball and tennis), because particular groups of muscles can be strained or torn by abruptly starting a forceful movement. Sudden falls are another common cause of injury, since you tend to extend your arm automatically to break a fall; the arm then bears the full weight of the body, often resulting in a fracture or a dislocation.

Injuries to the upper limbs include damage to the shoulder, arm, elbow, forearm, wrist, hand, and fingers.

## SHOULDER INJURIES

**Twisting and stretching injuries**
*Muscle and tendon strains are the most common shoulder injuries. They are caused by twisting the shoulder during a fall, overstretching one of the muscles, or repeating a specific shoulder movement (such as a tennis serve or a baseball pitch) many times.*

The shoulder joint is the most mobile joint in the body and has the widest range of motion. It is a ball-and-socket joint between the rounded head of the arm bone (the humerus) and the smooth depression (the glenoid fossa) in the shoulder blade (the scapula). The outer end of the collarbone (the clavicle) is attached to the top of the shoulder by ligaments; numerous muscles and tendons allow a wide range of motion.

Injuries to the supporting structures of the shoulder are common in sports. The exact area of pain and tenderness along with the movements that cause or aggravate the pain depend on which muscle or tendon has been damaged.

Treatment of a shoulder strain (overstretching a muscle) usually involves a few days of rest and, if necessary, treatment with an anti-inflammatory drug such as aspirin. Surgery is sometimes used to repair a torn tendon or a torn rotator cuff (a reinforcing structure around the shoulder made of muscles, tendons, and other fibers).

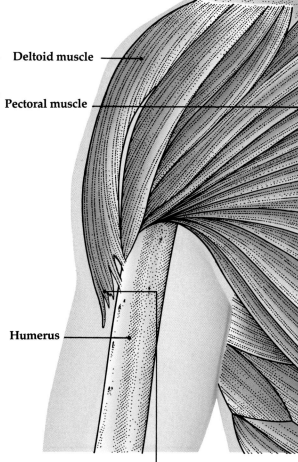

Deltoid muscle

Pectoral muscle

Humerus

**Muscle strains**
A strain of one of the muscles of the shoulder at the point where it attaches to the humerus may result from a repeated shoulder movement, as can occur when swimming the backstroke or lifting weights. If the tear is complete, it usually requires surgical repair.

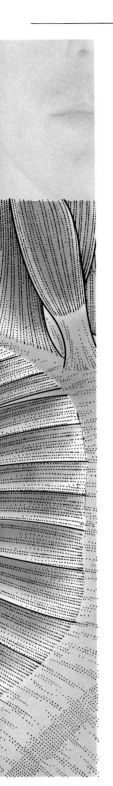

**Bursitis**
Inflammation of a bursa (one of the fluid-filled sacs that cushion the shoulder tendons from the bones) is caused by injury or by repetitive movement of the shoulder joint. Treatment involves rest followed by gentle exercise. Anti-inflammatory drugs such as aspirin are often recommended.

**Rotator cuff problems**
A common cause of shoulder pain is strain of the rotator cuff. The pain occurs when the arm is moved away from the side of the body. It is caused by an inflamed tendon rubbing against the acromion (the part of the shoulder blade nearest the joint). Rupture of the rotator cuff may occur during a heavy lift, a powerful throw, or a heavy fall on the shoulder.

Scapula

Clavicle

Acromioclavicular joint

Acromion

Bursa

Rotator cuff

**Synovitis**
Excessive shoulder exercise, or any shoulder injury, may lead to synovitis, a painful inflammation of the joint lining and surrounding tissues. An anti-inflammatory medication may be necessary to relieve the inflammation.

**Dislocations**
Both the acromioclavicular joint and the shoulder joint can be partially or totally dislocated as a result of a fall or a severe collision during contact sports. Treatment involves manipulating the joint back into position and immobilizing it until healing is complete. Occasionally, surgery is necessary to stabilize the joint, especially if the dislocation occurs more than once.

**Fractures**
Fractures around the shoulder may involve the clavicle, scapula, or head of the humerus. These fractures may be caused by a fall or by a severe blow. X-rays are taken to confirm the break. Among other considerations, treatment depends on the site of the fracture.

While you are recovering from a shoulder muscle or tendon strain, it is important to try to identify the movement that caused the injury so that you can avoid performing that move or modify it when you begin exercising again. Recurrent tendon strains can lead to persistent pain and stiffness that may require surgical treatment.

The bones and joints of the shoulder are also prone to injury from falls and collisions. Injuries can include partial or complete dislocation of the shoulder joint, as well as fractures of the clavicle, scapula, or the head of the humerus. Tendinitis (inflammation of a tendon), synovitis (inflammation of the joint lining), and bursitis (inflammation of one of the fluid-filled sacs cushioning the shoulder tendons) are shoulder problems that also occur frequently.

## UPPER ARM INJURIES

There is only one bone in the upper arm, the humerus. At its upper end, the humerus joins the scapula at the shoulder joint; at its lower end it forms part of the elbow joint. Pain and tenderness in the upper arm are usually caused by overstretching or overusing one of the muscles. However, pain may also be "referred" from the shoulder joint to the middle portion of your arm.

### Nerve damage and fractures

Other causes of pain in your upper arm include injuries to the neck (see page 90) or shoulder that have damaged one of the nerves that pass into the arm. Pain of this type may be caused by a disc problem in the neck that is exerting pressure on a nerve leading to the arm. In football a "stinger" may result when a player lands on the turf with his or her head going one way and the shoulder going the other, causing a momentary stretching of the nerves (this is usually a brief injury). Occasionally, a severe blow or fall causes a fracture of the humerus.

### TYPES OF INJURIES TO THE UPPER ARM

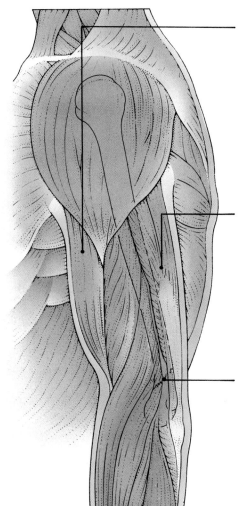

**Biceps strain**
The biceps is the main muscle at the front of the upper arm. Lengthy or repeated contraction of the biceps, which occurs in weight lifting, may cause inflammation and, occasionally, rupture of the muscle.

**Triceps pain**
The triceps is the main muscle at the back of the upper arm. Pain in this area may be caused by overstretching, which can occur when taking an excessive swing during a backhand shot in tennis.

**Humerus fractures**
Sports injuries that affect the humerus include fractures and dislocations of the shoulder joint between the humerus and the scapula. If the humerus is fractured at its upper end, it is usually immobilized in a sling for several weeks. If the lower end is fractured, a plaster cast may be required. Surgery may also be considered.

**Rowing**
*Rowing is an excellent form of aerobic exercise. However, as in any other activity in which you exert yourself against a form of resistance, start gradually and allow your arm, stomach, and back muscles to recover for a day between sessions until you build up strength.*

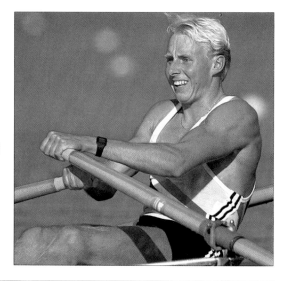

# CASE HISTORY
## RECURRENT SHOULDER DISLOCATION

S HARON DISLOCATED **her right shoulder 2 years ago while skiing. She dislocated it a second time while roller-skating. On both occasions the shoulder was manipulated back into position at a hospital and immobilized in a sling for 3 weeks. One morning, Sharon quickly stretched back her arm to put on her coat and dislocated her shoulder again. Her husband drove her to the emergency room.**

**PERSONAL DETAILS**
**Name** Sharon Eckstein
**Age** 36
**Occupation** Laboratory technician
**Family** Her father died in an accident; her mother is well. She has one sister, who is healthy. Sharon has two healthy children.

### MEDICAL BACKGROUND
Apart from recurrent earaches as a child, and her two previous shoulder injuries, Sharon has never had any serious health problems.

### THE CONSULTATION
By the time Sharon reaches the emergency room, her shoulder has popped back into position. But after taking Sharon's history, the emergency room doctor advises her to see an orthopedist soon. Because this dislocation was caused by a simple motion she makes every day – as opposed to a forceful injury – Sharon may require further treatment for her shoulder. The orthopedist tells Sharon that the previous dislocations have damaged the structures around her shoulder that keep the joint in place. The doctor explains that dislocation weakens the shoulder by stretching and tearing the joint capsule (covering) and the surrounding ligaments and tendons. In addition, damage to the cartilage that lines the rim of the socket on one side of the scapula, along with scraping of the bone on the head of the humerus, may have made the joint even more unstable. It is common after two dislocations for the shoulder to be left permanently weakened, so that even ordinary movements can cause a dislocation. The specialist recommends that Sharon undergo surgery to have the joint stabilized.

### THE OPERATION
Sharon has an operation to strengthen the supporting structures around her shoulder joint. The surgery is performed while Sharon is under general anesthesia; the operation takes about 1 hour. The tendons are tightened and repositioned, and the muscles and skin are then stitched back into position. A dressing is placed over the shoulder and upper arm, and a thick cotton pad is put in her armpit. Sharon's shoulder is then immobilized in a collar and cuff sling, with a bandage securing her arm against her body. Sharon stays in the hospital for a day.

### THE OUTCOME
After the operation, Sharon keeps her right arm immobilized for 4 weeks. The doctor then gives Sharon a program of progressively more strenuous exercises to help her move her shoulder freely and to strengthen the surrounding muscles. Sharon does the exercises regularly and, within 3 months, she reports no further problems. The doctor tells her that she can return to her normal activities.

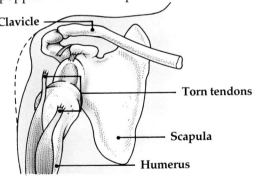

Clavicle
Torn tendons
Scapula
Humerus

**Dislocated shoulder**
*A dislocated shoulder occurs when the round end of the humerus slips out of its socket in the scapula. Sometimes, as in Sharon's case, torn tendons require surgery. A shoulder immobilizer (right) helps protect the joint after the operation.*

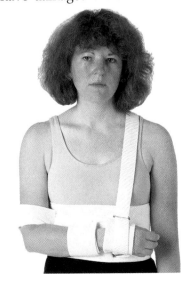

# INJURIES TO THE ELBOW AND FOREARM

The elbow joint, which allows the arm to bend or straighten and the forearm to rotate inward and outward, is a complex structure. It is important not only in sports but also in the performance of most everyday activities, such as dressing, bathing, and eating.

Elbow injuries often occur during sports that involve throwing. The injuries may be more serious than they appear. This is true particularly for children and for adolescents who may still be growing because their arm muscles are attached to areas of bone that are growing. These areas are much weaker than the adjacent bone and are therefore more vulnerable to injury. For this reason, children should not be allowed to pitch more than three innings of baseball every other day. Playing catch, however, does not cause a problem. If there seems to be any major problem with your child's elbow, such as loss of motion or being unable to straighten the elbow, talk to your child's doctor immediately.

The bones of the forearm are the radius and the ulna. They work in conjunction with one another. Injuries can involve one or both of the bones.

### Dislocated elbow
Dislocation of the elbow is rare. It usually occurs during contact sports such as football or activities that can lead to a fall, such as bicycling. After the dislocation has been confirmed with X-rays, the doctor manipulates the bones back into position and puts the elbow in a plaster cast.

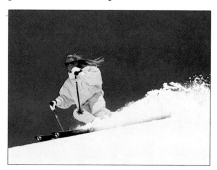

### Dislocated elbow in childhood
A less serious form of dislocation, which is common in children, involves the head of the radius being pulled forward as the arm is stretched out straight. Your doctor can easily manipulate this type of dislocation back into place by rotating the elbow.

## TYPES OF INJURIES TO THE ELBOW AND FOREARM

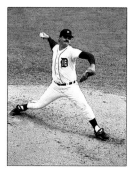

**Loose bodies (fragments of bone and cartilage)**
Repeated throwing movements or recurrent injury to the elbow may cause fragments of bone and cartilage to break off inside the joint. These loose bodies, which may or may not be apparent on X-rays, may lodge between the bones, preventing normal movement. Orthopedic surgery may be needed to remove these fragments from your joint; in some instances, the surgery can be done through an arthroscope (see page 111).

**Fracture of the head of the radius**
You may fracture the head of the radius if you stretch out your hand to break a fall and then fall heavily on the hand. If an X-ray shows that the bone has broken into several pieces, these fragments are usually removed by an operation.

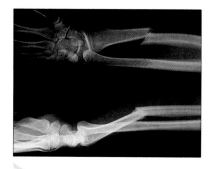

**Fractured forearm**
A fracture of one or both bones in the forearm may be caused by a fall or a direct blow. In the upper or middle third of the forearm the fracture can be treated with a cast alone. Sometimes the doctor manipulates the bones back into place and secures them with screws and a metal plate. The arm is then immobilized in plaster, with the elbow held at a right angle, for at least 6 weeks.

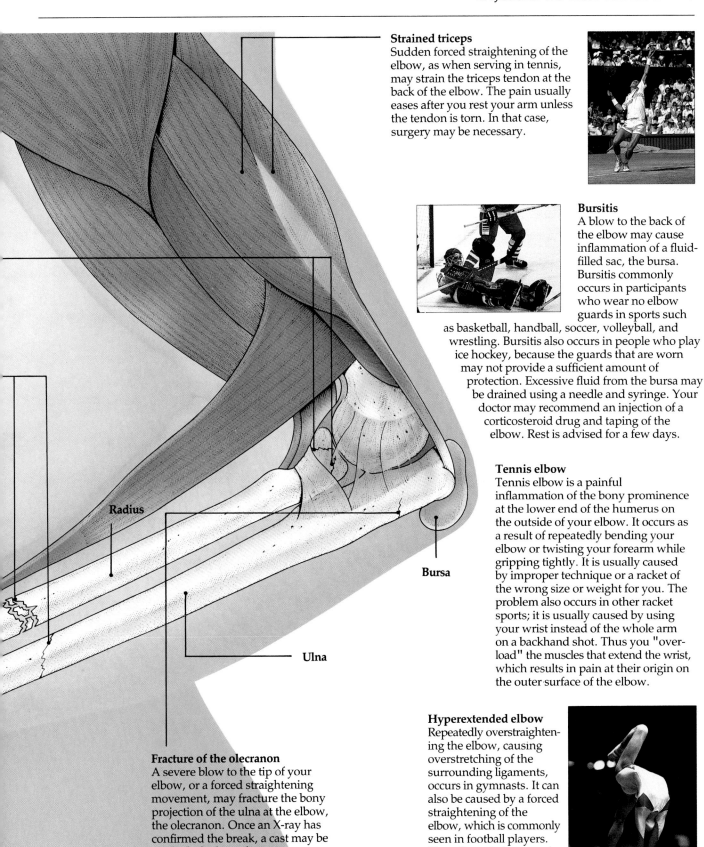

**Strained triceps**
Sudden forced straightening of the elbow, as when serving in tennis, may strain the triceps tendon at the back of the elbow. The pain usually eases after you rest your arm unless the tendon is torn. In that case, surgery may be necessary.

**Bursitis**
A blow to the back of the elbow may cause inflammation of a fluid-filled sac, the bursa. Bursitis commonly occurs in participants who wear no elbow guards in sports such as basketball, handball, soccer, volleyball, and wrestling. Bursitis also occurs in people who play ice hockey, because the guards that are worn may not provide a sufficient amount of protection. Excessive fluid from the bursa may be drained using a needle and syringe. Your doctor may recommend an injection of a corticosteroid drug and taping of the elbow. Rest is advised for a few days.

**Tennis elbow**
Tennis elbow is a painful inflammation of the bony prominence at the lower end of the humerus on the outside of your elbow. It occurs as a result of repeatedly bending your elbow or twisting your forearm while gripping tightly. It is usually caused by improper technique or a racket of the wrong size or weight for you. The problem also occurs in other racket sports; it is usually caused by using your wrist instead of the whole arm on a backhand shot. Thus you "overload" the muscles that extend the wrist, which results in pain at their origin on the outer surface of the elbow.

**Radius**

**Bursa**

**Ulna**

**Hyperextended elbow**
Repeatedly overstraightening the elbow, causing overstretching of the surrounding ligaments, occurs in gymnasts. It can also be caused by a forced straightening of the elbow, which is commonly seen in football players. Once the pain has eased, you may need to exercise to build up the muscles in your arm.

**Fracture of the olecranon**
A severe blow to the tip of your elbow, or a forced straightening movement, may fracture the bony projection of the ulna at the elbow, the olecranon. Once an X-ray has confirmed the break, a cast may be applied, the bone fragment may have to be reattached with a screw, or the triceps tendon may be stitched to another part of the ulna.

# Injuries to the inside of the elbow

Most elbow injuries occur to the outside or back of the elbow. Some, however, affect the inside of the elbow. A blow to the inside of the elbow may send a "pins-and-needles" sensation down your forearm into the fourth and fifth fingers of your hand. This odd feeling is caused by irritation of the ulnar nerve and has led to the term "funny bone." Rest usually eases the discomfort. However, in serious cases, especially if the sensation appears every time you exercise that elbow, surgery may be needed to move the nerve to a different part of the elbow.

**The elbow in tennis**
*Striking a tennis ball forcibly with "spin" or "cut" many times in a session causes not only inflammation of the outside of the elbow (tennis elbow), but it can also cause irritation of the ulnar nerve.*

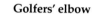

**Golfers' elbow**
*Golfers' elbow is a painful inflammation of the bony prominence at the lower end of the humerus. It is similar to tennis elbow except that it is on the inside of the joint. Golfers' elbow is caused by overworking the muscles on the front of the forearm, which bend your wrist and fingers downward. It can occur if golfers jar their elbows when they strike too far below a golf ball, hitting the ground.*

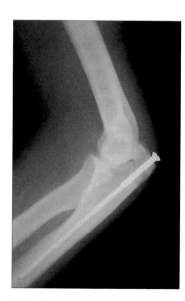

**Fracture of the tip of the elbow**
*The tip of the elbow (the olecranon) can be displaced and separated from the ulna in the forearm by a sudden blow. The displacement will not heal without treatment because the triceps tendon pulls the olecranon away from the ulna. To treat this injury, the doctor uses a screw to secure the displaced bone (left). A cast is used only in cases where the bone is not displaced or if the patient has a medical condition that prevents surgery.*

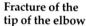
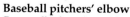

**Baseball pitchers' elbow**
*Repeatedly throwing with spin, as in baseball, may inflame the tendons on the inside of the elbow. Children and adolescents who overdo their pitching may get little leaguers' elbow, in which inflamed tendons pull away from the growing area of bone at the point where they attach.*

# INJURIES TO THE WRIST

The wrist has an intricate structure, with eight small carpal bones arranged in two rows of four. There are small joints between each pair of carpal bones, and the joints are bound together by ligaments running around and across the back and front of your wrist.

Your wrist movements are controlled by the muscles in your forearm. The tendons of these muscles pass over the wrist bones and attach to the bones in the hand. The highly mobile wrist joint allows the hand to move up and down through an angle of 180 degrees, from side to side through an angle of 30 degrees, or in a circular fashion.

## Common injuries

Ligament sprain (an injury in which the fibers are partially torn) is a common wrist injury. It may be caused by a fall on an outstretched hand that forces your wrist beyond its normal range of movement, by a jarring force (such as catching a fast pitch in baseball), or by repeated overstretching, which can occur when practicing a tennis shot using poor technique. The wrist should be taped and rested for a few days.

Tenosynovitis is another common wrist injury. It is a painful inflammation of the tendons that occurs as a result of any repeated wrist action. In rowing, it may be caused by gripping an oar handle too tightly, or by using a handle of the wrong size.

**Contact sports and injuries**
*Sprains and dislocations of the wrist occur in many sports in which falls and repeated trauma are common, such as ice hockey (left), volleyball, basketball, and football. The injured athlete should rest immediately and apply an ice pack to the injury. A doctor should be consulted; any undiagnosed and untreated fracture or dislocation may not heal properly.*

## TYPES OF INJURIES TO THE WRIST

**Sprained wrist**
A wrist sprain is the most common wrist injury. Occasionally, the sprain causes a swelling of a tendon sheath, known as a ganglion, on the back of the wrist. This swelling moves when you move your wrist and occasionally becomes painful. You may need an injection of a corticosteroid drug or minor surgery.

**Tendons**

**Median nerve**

**Carpal tunnel**

**Tendon sheaths**

**Carpal tunnel syndrome**
Any wrist injury that leads to swelling of the tissues surrounding the median nerve (see above) or inflammation of the tendons of the wrist from prolonged gripping can cause carpal tunnel syndrome. This causes pain, numbness, and tingling in the thumb, index finger, and middle fingers. Occasionally, the doctor must put your wrist in a splint or give you a corticosteroid drug. In rare cases, surgery is required.

**Tenosynovitis**
Tenosynovitis is a painful inflammation of the tendon linings and is a common wrist injury in any sport in which repeated wrist movements or a powerful grip are required. It often causes swelling over the tendons. You may hear a crackle or experience a grating sensation when you move your wrist.

In racket sports, tenosynovitis may be caused by a faulty grip or a racket handle of the wrong size. The pain is usually worse when you try to grip any object. Treatment calls for resting the wrist in a splint or taping it. Occasionally, the wrist is placed in a plaster cast.

If your symptoms do not improve, you may ultimately need surgery to relieve the pressure on the inflamed tendon. Once you have recovered, it is important to try to determine the cause of your injury so you can change your performance or technique if necessary.

## Fractures

A fall onto your hand may fracture the scaphoid bone (one of the carpal bones in the wrist) or the bones of the lower end of your forearm (the radius or the ulna). A fracture of the forearm causes pain, swelling, tenderness, and deformity of the wrist. A Colles fracture is a type of break in which the bone fragment is forced upward and backward over the rest of the radius and the tip of the ulna is broken. The doctor manipulates the bones back into position and immobilizes them in a plaster cast for about 6 weeks.

A stress fracture of the lower end of the radius may occur in gymnasts because of repeated vaulting (i.e., twisting as they shift their entire body weight over the wrist).

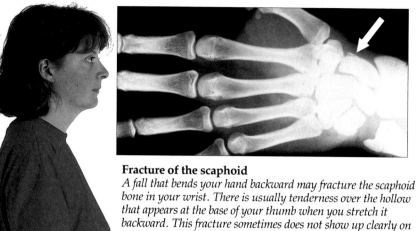

**Fracture of the scaphoid**
*A fall that bends your hand backward may fracture the scaphoid bone in your wrist. There is usually tenderness over the hollow that appears at the base of your thumb when you stretch it backward. This fracture sometimes does not show up clearly on an X-ray until several days later. If you have pain in your hand after a fall and there is tenderness over the scaphoid (see above), you should have an X-ray. If the scaphoid is fractured, your thumb, hand, wrist, and forearm must be immobilized in a plaster cast for several weeks or the bone may not heal properly. Arthritis may develop after this injury.*

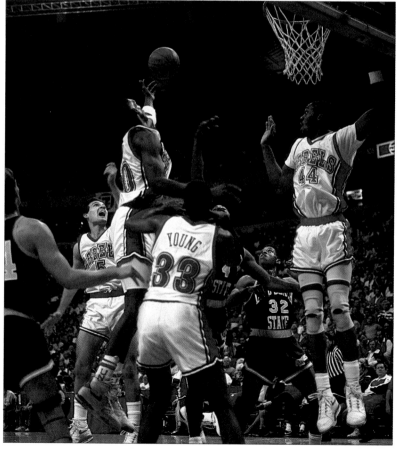

**Catching and throwing**
*Injuries to the hands and fingers frequently occur in sports such as basketball or softball that involve catching or throwing a ball.*

# INJURIES TO THE HANDS AND FINGERS

Your hand is most frequently injured in sports that involve catching or throwing a ball, or holding a racket, bat, or stick. Any abrasion or cut on the hand should be cleaned carefully to prevent infection. If a wound becomes inflamed or drains pus, consult your doctor to determine whether the wound should be drained further or you need an antibiotic.

## Ligament injuries

If you twist your finger awkwardly while catching or throwing a ball, you may sprain a ligament. This is a particularly common injury in basketball and football players, but usually there is only minor damage. The finger is treated by taping it to the adjacent finger for about 2 weeks; you may then be advised to start bending and straightening the finger. If a ligament in your finger is completely torn, the finger joint may have to be immobilized in a plaster cast or repaired surgically. Even a minor ligament injury may cause swelling and stiffness that could last for several months.

## TYPES OF HAND INJURIES

**Dislocated finger**
Dislocation of a finger usually involves the little finger or thumb and frequently occurs when you catch a ball awkwardly. Occasionally, your doctor can reposition the joint by pulling sharply on the end of the finger; this should be attempted only by a trained professional. It is mandatory to have an X-ray to ensure that there is no fracture of the finger.

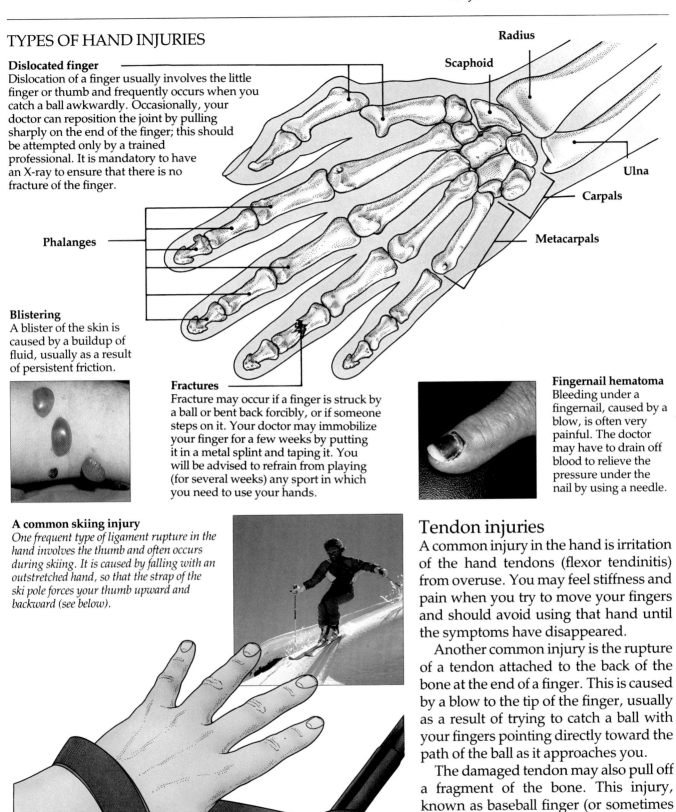

Radius

Scaphoid

Ulna

Carpals

Metacarpals

Phalanges

**Blistering**
A blister of the skin is caused by a buildup of fluid, usually as a result of persistent friction.

**Fractures**
Fracture may occur if a finger is struck by a ball or bent back forcibly, or if someone steps on it. Your doctor may immobilize your finger for a few weeks by putting it in a metal splint and taping it. You will be advised to refrain from playing (for several weeks) any sport in which you need to use your hands.

**Fingernail hematoma**
Bleeding under a fingernail, caused by a blow, is often very painful. The doctor may have to drain off blood to relieve the pressure under the nail by using a needle.

**A common skiing injury**
*One frequent type of ligament rupture in the hand involves the thumb and often occurs during skiing. It is caused by falling with an outstretched hand, so that the strap of the ski pole forces your thumb upward and backward (see below).*

**Ruptured ligament**

## Tendon injuries

A common injury in the hand is irritation of the hand tendons (flexor tendinitis) from overuse. You may feel stiffness and pain when you try to move your fingers and should avoid using that hand until the symptoms have disappeared.

Another common injury is the rupture of a tendon attached to the back of the bone at the end of a finger. This is caused by a blow to the tip of the finger, usually as a result of trying to catch a ball with your fingers pointing directly toward the path of the ball as it approaches you.

The damaged tendon may also pull off a fragment of the bone. This injury, known as baseball finger (or sometimes mallet finger), will prevent you from straightening your finger as you normally would. Occasionally, the finger will remain bent for a while, but you should not have any trouble using it.

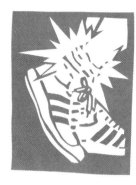

# INJURIES TO THE LOWER LIMBS

YOUR LEGS, CONNECTED TO YOUR torso by powerful muscles and tendons at your stable hip joints, carry the weight of your body. During a fall or awkward twisting motion, however, much of the weight may be shifted to a knee or to an ankle, causing strained muscles, torn ligaments, and even broken bones. The legs are also vulnerable to a range of injuries during contact sports caused by kicks, tackling, and sudden turns when your foot is flat on the floor.

Lower limb injuries during exercise include damage to the foot, ankle, leg, knee, thigh, hip, and groin.

## INJURIES TO THE FOOT

The foot is an intricate structure consisting of 26 individual bones and related muscles, tendons, and ligaments. The bones vary in size from the large heel bone (the calcaneus) to the tiny bones (the phalanges) that form the toes.

The foot must support the weight of your body and also act as a springboard when you walk or run. The heels and the balls of the feet take most of the impact. The skin on the sole of the foot is usually thicker in these areas. There is also a strong layer of protective tissue, the plantar fascia, just beneath the skin on

## TYPES OF FOOT INJURIES

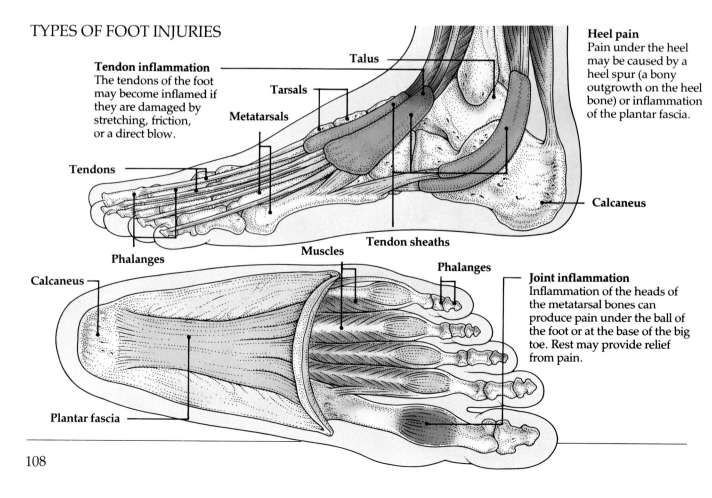

**Tendon inflammation**
The tendons of the foot may become inflamed if they are damaged by stretching, friction, or a direct blow.

Tendons

Phalanges

Calcaneus

Plantar fascia

Talus

Tarsals

Metatarsals

Tendon sheaths

Muscles

Phalanges

**Heel pain**
Pain under the heel may be caused by a heel spur (a bony outgrowth on the heel bone) or inflammation of the plantar fascia.

Calcaneus

**Joint inflammation**
Inflammation of the heads of the metatarsal bones can produce pain under the ball of the foot or at the base of the big toe. Rest may provide relief from pain.

## SPRAINED ANKLE

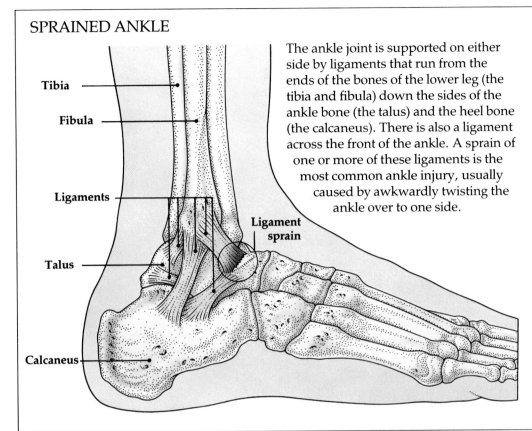

Tibia

Fibula

Ligaments

Talus

Calcaneus

Ligament sprain

The ankle joint is supported on either side by ligaments that run from the ends of the bones of the lower leg (the tibia and fibula) down the sides of the ankle bone (the talus) and the heel bone (the calcaneus). There is also a ligament across the front of the ankle. A sprain of one or more of these ligaments is the most common ankle injury, usually caused by awkwardly twisting the ankle over to one side.

**Broken ankle**
*It is difficult to tell whether an ankle injury is simply a sprained ligament, or whether a bone has been broken, too. A sprain can cause just as much pain and swelling as a broken bone, and it may be impossible to bear weight on the ankle even if it is not broken. After any painful injury to your ankle, it is a good idea to have an X-ray.*

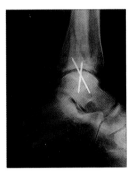

the sole of the foot, that covers the underlying muscles and tendons. A complex network of blood vessels and nerves runs through the tissues on both the sole and the top of the foot.

The most common injury to the foot is a sprained ligament. This can be caused by a sudden sharp twist, an awkward landing, or repeated overstretching caused by a poor choice of shoes or substandard technique. Pain across the top of the foot may be caused by an inflammation of the tendon linings resulting from a direct blow, persistent overstretching, or friction from your shoes.

Pain in the ball of the foot is often caused by inflammation of the heads of the bones that form the main body of the foot (the metatarsals). This pain may be brought on by wearing shoes of the wrong size or of poor quality. For all injuries of the foot it is important to determine whether you might prevent a recurrence by switching to different shoes. Sometimes a metatarsal bar in a

shoe shifts the weight toward the heel and relieves the symptoms eventually.

## INJURIES TO THE ANKLE

The ankle joint absorbs a lot of jarring when you run, change direction, or jump (especially on hard surfaces). The most common injury to the joint during exercise is a sprained ankle, which occurs when your foot turns over on its edge and the ligaments of the foot are stretched. Ligaments in the ankle may be sprained if you trip while running.

Damage to the ligaments in the ankle is usually no more serious than a sprain, but the ligament may be torn completely. If this occurs, the ankle is likely to become unstable. Treatment of a more serious sprain involves immobilizing the joint in a cast or splint or surgical repair. Repeated injury to the ankle can lead to chronic instability and later to arthritic changes. Abnormal scarring may then block the free movement of the joint.

**The ankle as a pivot**
*Ankle injuries are common in those who play tennis, basketball, or football because these sports demand jumping and rapid changes of direction. Players may land awkwardly and turn their ankles sideways.*

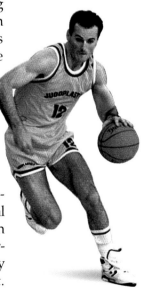

# INJURIES TO THE KNEE

The knee is one of the more mobile joints in your body. It is a hinged and flexible joint that allows bending movements and rapid changes of direction, while providing the stability needed to hold the leg in an upright standing position. However, the knee is highly susceptible to injury caused by sudden twisting or bending, and such movements commonly damage the cartilage or ligaments surrounding the knee joint.

**Strain or rupture of a ligament**
Damage to a knee ligament is one of the most common injuries in sports. Injury to the medial ligament is more common than damage to the lateral. Cruciate ligament injury may be the most common of all. Minor strain causes pain, tenderness, and swelling. If the medial or cruciate ligaments are ruptured, the stability of the knee is affected.

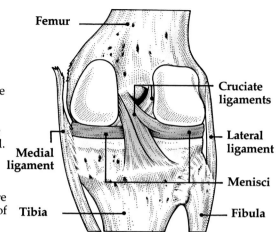

**Injury to the knee cartilage**
Damage to the cartilage inside the knee joint is very common. If healing is inadequate, the torn cartilage may need to be removed.

## TYPES OF KNEE INJURIES

**Runners' knee**
Runners or joggers are susceptible to at least two types of inflammation known as runners' knee. Inflammation causes pain of the iliotibial tract, a fibrous band that runs down the outside of the knee from the buttock muscles to the tibia. Inflammation of the tendon of the kneecap (the patella), which attaches the kneecap to the shin, is also called runners' knee.

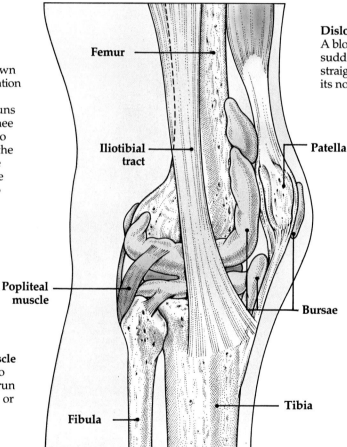

**Dislocated kneecap**
A blow to the side of the knee or a sudden twist when the knee is almost straight may force the kneecap out of its normal position.

**Chondromalacia patellae**
In this disorder, damage to the joint surface at the back of the patella causes pain behind the kneecap. Doctors think the problem occurs because the patella is tilted at an abnormal angle. The tilting may be caused by muscle imbalance around the knee.

**Strain of the popliteal muscle**
Long-distance runners who run downhill extensively, run on roads with steep banks, or have an abnormal foot alignment may strain the popliteal muscle located at the back of the knee.

**Bursitis**
Repeated pressure, strain, or a blow to the knee may cause inflammation of one of the fluid-filled sacs (bursae) surrounding the knee joint. Wrestlers are prone to bursitis in the front of the knee because of the pressure that they place on their knees.

**Osteoarthritis**
Repeated injury to the knee can lead to osteoarthritis, a disease that causes pain, swelling, and stiffness of the joints. Osteoarthritis is characterized by degeneration of the cartilage that lines the joints and by the formation of bony growths.

You can generally estimate the severity of a knee injury by the speed at which swelling occurs afterward. Rapid swelling is usually caused by bleeding inside the joint and may be traced to a tear in a cruciate ligament (one of the two ligaments in each knee that forms a cross) or cartilage. A doctor usually attempts to remove the blood from inside the joint with a needle and syringe. Other symptoms of a cartilage injury include instability or locking of the knee in one position. Locking occurs when a loose fragment of cartilage becomes trapped between the surfaces of the knee joint.

If swelling does not appear until at least 12 hours after the injury, damage to the knee is probably less severe. Slow swelling is usually caused by an increased production of synovial fluid as a result of inflammation of the membrane lining the capsule of the knee joint. This type of swelling, known as synovitis, may develop after any type of ligament injury, a small tear in the joint capsule, or a small tear of the cartilage.

**A knee injury in the making**
*A common cause of injury in sports is a sudden twist of the knee while it is bent and taking the full weight of the body. This stress is likely to tear a cartilage and commonly occurs in soccer, basketball, and football players and in those who ski. Strengthening the leg muscles helps prevent this injury.*

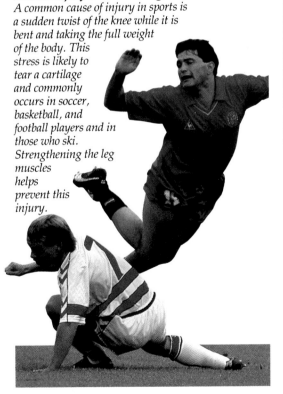

# SURGICAL PROCEDURES
## MENISCECTOMY (REMOVAL OF KNEE CARTILAGE)

**M**ENISCECTOMY **is used to remove part or all of the damaged knee cartilage (meniscus). The operation is often performed using an arthroscope – a small tubular viewing instrument inserted into the knee. Meniscectomy is avoided whenever possible because it may increase the risk of osteoarthritis. That risk must be balanced against the dangers of leaving a damaged meniscus inside the knee, disrupting normal function.**

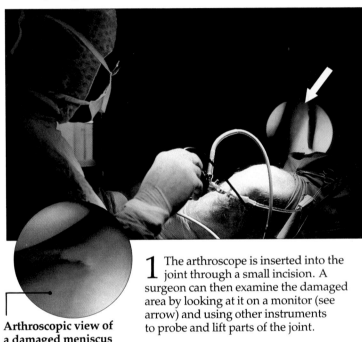

**Arthroscopic view of a damaged meniscus**

1 The arthroscope is inserted into the joint through a small incision. A surgeon can then examine the damaged area by looking at it on a monitor (see arrow) and using other instruments to probe and lift parts of the joint.

2 The damaged cartilage is removed using instruments passed into the knee through a small separate incision. If any additional surgery on the joint is needed, it is done next. After surgery, the incisions are closed with one suture or an adhesive strip and the patient goes home the same day.

**Arthroscope (viewing instrument)**

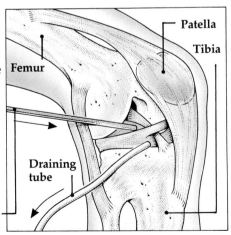

**Patella**

**Tibia**

**Femur**

**Draining tube**

# LEG AND CALF INJURIES

## TYPES OF LEG INJURIES

Injuries of the leg are usually caused by overexertion. Some people develop strains of the muscles and tendons in the leg as a result of running on hard surfaces or wearing worn-out shoes or the wrong shoes for a particular activity. People who have an abnormal foot alignment that causes their feet to turn inward or who run on the outside edges of their soles are also susceptible to leg injuries. Corrective devices, worn inside the shoe, may be used to reduce the risk of injury caused by these foot problems.

If pain develops in your leg when you run and the pain is worse when you move your foot, consider having your shoes, running style, and training routine evaluated to determine the cause of the problem. Maintaining fitness by swimming, cycling, or workouts at a gym, rather than by exercises involving running, greatly reduces the amount of stress that you place on your legs.

**Fractures**
A sudden blow to the leg or a severe injury to the ankle may fracture the tibia or fibula. Your doctor may apply a cast to such fractures, but sometimes they require surgery to secure the fragments in place with nails, plates, or screws.

**Stress fracture**
Repeated stress may lead to a small crack in the tibia or fibula. Stress fractures usually develop as a result of running or working out on hard surfaces.

**Achilles tendinitis**
Minor injuries to the Achilles tendon are common. Inflammation of the tendon may result from a session of intensive training, especially if it involves running uphill. Pain may also occur as the result of changing running surfaces or breaking in a new pair of shoes. Shoes with high counters (heel tabs) on the back of the shoe (so-called tendon protectors) may cause Achilles tendinitis if there is a lot of friction between the counter and the tendon.

**Strain of the calf muscle**
A tearing of part of the inner calf muscle may be caused by sudden stretching, by landing awkwardly on the toes, or by doing an exercise to which you are not accustomed. Calf muscle strain is more common in older people.

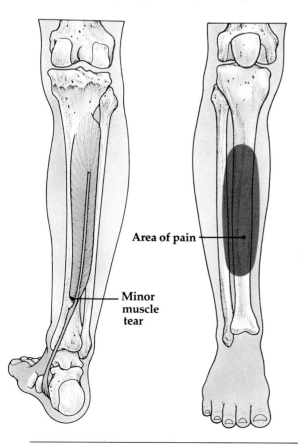

**Area of pain**

**Minor muscle tear**

**Shin splints**
Aching pain that develops at the front of the leg is referred to as shin splints and may have a number of causes. A minor tear of a muscle, inflammation of the periosteum (fibrous covering) of the tibia, increased pressure in the anterior tibial compartment of the leg, or a stress fracture may cause shin splints.

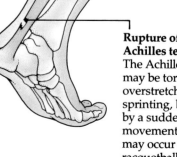

**Rupture of the Achilles tendon**
The Achilles tendon may be torn by sudden overstretching during sprinting, by jumping, by a sudden movement (such as may occur during racquetball), or by a direct blow. If the tendon is torn apart completely, surgical repair is usually necessary.

# INJURIES TO THE HIP AND GROIN

The hip is the largest joint in your body. The round head of the thigh bone, the femur, fits snugly into the acetabulum, a shallow, rounded cavity on the outer wall of your pelvis. Hip injuries are uncommon in sports because the hip joint is highly stable and considerable force is required to dislocate it. While shoulder dislocations are common, hip dislocations usually occur only in accidents that result from activities such as auto racing.

More vulnerable, however, is the groin, a web of ligaments and muscles lying between the lower part of your abdominal wall and the upper part of the thigh. The inguinal canal passes through both sides of this part of the lower abdominal wall; the canal is the channel through which the testes pass before birth and which contains the spermatic cord in men and a ligament in women. Hernia (a protrusion of tissue or part of an internal organ through a weakness in a muscular wall) frequently occurs in this area because the canal contributes to the potential muscular weakness.

### REFERRED PAIN

Pain felt in your hip may originate from an injury in your back, groin, or knee; similarly, a hip injury may cause pain in those areas. Or the pain from a hip disorder may appear in the front of your thigh. This pain is called referred pain and is taken into account when diagnosing a hip problem.

## TYPES OF INJURIES TO THE HIP AND GROIN

**Hip sprain**
The hip may be sprained by a twisting injury that damages the ligaments or causes inflammation of the capsule that encloses the joint. Moving your hip becomes painful and stiff and you may limp slightly when you walk.

**Buttock strain**
Pain on the outside of your hip may be caused by a strain of the gluteal (buttock) muscle at the point where it attaches to the upper end of your thigh bone. This injury most commonly occurs during long-distance running.

**Hip joint**
The ball-and-socket structure of the joint between the femur and the pelvis accounts for much of the hip's stability.

**Pelvic bone**

**Acetabulum**

**Femur**

**Gluteal muscle**

**Adductor muscle injury**
Injury to the adductor muscles is the most common cause of pain in the groin. Pain that persists after rest may be caused by a small fragment of the pelvic bone that may have been pulled off, or by a severe tear. An anti-inflammatory drug such as aspirin or an injection of a corticosteroid drug is sometimes enough to reduce the pain. However, occasionally the injury needs surgical repair.

**Adductor muscles**

**Bursa**

**Groin pull**
The term "groin pull" describes pain and tenderness in the groin, usually caused by overstretching a muscle while you are running or moving abruptly during exercise. The muscles commonly affected are the adductors and the rectus femoris.

**Fracture of the neck of the femur**
In rare cases, a fall that occurs while someone is traveling at high speeds, such as can occur while skiing or cycling, can cause a fracture of the neck of the femur. Long-distance running may cause a stress fracture in some people.

**Bursitis**
Pain in the outer part of your hip may be caused by bursitis, which is inflammation of a fluid-filled sac (a bursa) that lies under the tendons running across your hip. Hip bursitis may result from a direct blow or from friction caused by an abnormal style of running.

113

## INJURIES TO THE THIGH

Your thigh contains the largest bone in your body, the femur, which has a rounded head at its upper end, an angled neck, a long thick shaft, and two bony prominences called condyles at its lower end. The head of the femur forms the hip joint with the outside of the pelvis, and the condyles (rounded ends of a bone) are part of the knee joint.

### The quadriceps muscles

The quadriceps muscles, which make up the bulk of the muscle at the front of your thigh, may be injured by a direct kick or blow. This type of injury may cause bleeding within the muscles. The quadriceps muscle may also be torn by overstretching your leg or by having your movement suddenly blocked just when you are straightening your knee (as when you are tackled at the moment you kick a ball). These injuries may cause tenderness, pain, and swelling at the site of the damage; bruising often appears a few days after the injury.

In most cases of quadriceps injury, the damage heals naturally within a few days. It is important to rest for at least a couple of days before you begin exercising the leg muscles again. You should do very gradually any exercises to restore thigh strength that involve a full range of knee movement. Occasionally, a severe quadriceps muscle tear requires surgery.

If an injury to one of the muscles in your thigh does not improve within a few weeks, and pain prevents you from exercising, it may be that a small fragment of bone has been pulled off the pelvis at the point where a muscle is attached. This problem must be treated by a doctor.

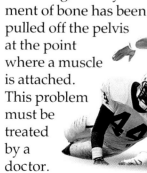

## TYPES OF THIGH INJURIES

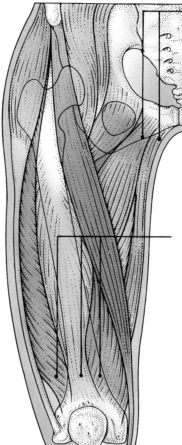

**Strain of the adductor muscles**
Pain on the inside of your thigh may be caused by a strain or tear in one of the adductor muscles. These muscles may be strained during a long horse ride, or while running if you have an abnormal foot alignment in which your foot turns outward each time it touches the ground. The adductors may be torn if your leg is forced away from the torso during a fall or tackle, or if you take too long a stride when running uphill. Performing a split in gymnastics can also injure these muscles.

**Strain of the quadriceps muscles**
Repeated extreme contractions of the quadriceps muscles, which may occur during prolonged running, cycling uphill, or repeated squat thrust exercises, can cause a strain. The muscle damage is usually at the top of the thigh or just above the knee. Gentle stretching exercises can be started soon after this type of injury.

**Strain of the hamstring muscles**
A sudden, severe pain in the area of the three hamstring muscles at the back of your thigh is usually caused by exercising without a warm-up. The hamstrings may also be strained by repeated overstretching, especially if you have become tired toward the end of a training session. In this case the pain comes on gradually rather than suddenly. Occasionally, a kick to the back of the thigh tears a hamstring.

**Fracture of the femur**
A break in the femur is a rare occurrence in sports, although a severe blow to the thigh or to just above the knee can damage this large bone.

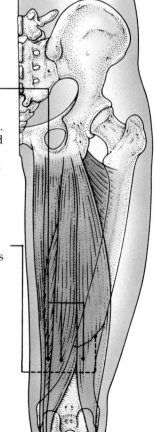

**Football**
*Perhaps the definitive contact sport, football carries a high risk of thigh and/or leg injury.*

# CASE HISTORY
# PERSISTENT GROIN PAIN

**M**IKE FIRST NOTICED PAIN in his left groin about 2 months ago. The pain got progressively worse each time he exercised. Mike stopped playing racquetball for 5 weeks, hoping that the pain would disappear, but it returned as soon as he started exercising again. While playing soccer with his son in the backyard, a searing pain shot through his groin the first time he kicked the ball. Mike decided to make an appointment to see his doctor as quickly as possible.

### PERSONAL DETAILS
**Name** Mike Vandlik
**Age** 39
**Occupation** Truck driver
**Family** Both parents are well. One brother has asthma.

## MEDICAL BACKGROUND
Mike last saw his doctor 3 years ago for a physical examination needed for his job. He considers himself healthy and in good shape, but would like to lose a few pounds.

## THE CONSULTATION
Describing the pain in his left groin, Mike tells his doctor that rest gave him only slight relief. At first he had attributed the pain to a muscle strain that had occurred while swimming. But his groin now feels sensitive to movement, especially when he must stand for long periods, and he is concerned by the new pain that he felt when he kicked the soccer ball. During a physical examination, the doctor finds that Mike's left groin is highly sensitive. Although there is no visible swelling in the groin, the doctor can feel a small protuberance when he pushes a finger up through the side of the scrotum into the entrance of the inguinal canal, which runs through the groin.

## THE DIAGNOSIS
Mike learns that he has a small IN-GUINAL HERNIA. Part of the peritoneum, the lining of the abdominal cavity, is protruding down through a weak spot in the muscle wall of his abdomen. This weak area is located at the point where the inguinal canal passes across a ligament. Mike's swelling can easily be pushed back into his abdomen. The doctor finds no indication that a loop of bowel has been trapped inside the hernia and, because Mike wants to return to his regular exercise routine, he recommends that Mike have an inguinal hernia repair operation.

## THE TREATMENT
The doctor makes an incision directly over the hernia and the protruding area of the inner part of the abdomen is pressed back into its correct position. The weakened area in Mike's abdominal wall is then repaired and reinforced.

## THE OUTLOOK
Following his operation, which was an outpatient procedure, Mike goes home to rest in bed for a day or two. Even a short walk is painful at first. However, once the wound begins to heal and the pain eases, the doctor gives Mike a program of rehabilitation exercises to help him recover and reduce the risk of a recurrence.

**Diagnosing a hernia**
*After hearing Mike's account of the pain in his lower abdomen, the doctor tells him that he may have an inguinal hernia.*

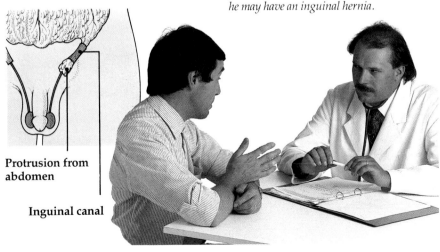

**Protrusion from abdomen**

**Inguinal canal**

# CHAPTER SIX

# RECOVERING FROM AN INJURY

## INTRODUCTION

## REHABILITATION AFTER AN INJURY

## REHABILITATION EXERCISES

IF YOU PARTICIPATE in exercise or sports regularly and are eager to keep your body in good condition, an injury may cause you special frustration. You may wonder whether you can exercise the uninjured parts of your body while the injury heals (the answer is yes), and you may wonder how long recovery might take. With a few more serious injuries, you may even be concerned about whether your injury will permanently affect your physical condition or your ability to perform in your chosen exercise program or sport. In most cases, you can make a complete recovery from exercise-related injuries, and you can return to your previous activities without major problems. The key is to fit your rehabilitation program to your injury and personal habits. Some people make the mistake of returning abruptly to their previous level of activity as soon as they can after injury. This carries a high risk of recurrence of the original injury or another injury caused by your inability to coordinate muscular activity as well as you need to. If you have such a recurrence, you may wonder if the injury will be a problem for life, but this is not necessarily the case. What you need is a sensible and gradual program of recovery and rehabilitation. In the first section of this chapter, REHABILITATION AFTER AN INJURY, you will find information about the kinds of rehabilitation and care that you may need after an injury. The healing process that your tissues undergo to recover from an injury is described, along with the steps that you can take to facilitate your own recovery. It is important to call your doctor after an injury if there is any question as to how severe it is, so that you can be certain about the nature of the injury and about the appropriate treatment program. The first step, at least for many minor injuries, is the time-tested first aid series called RICE – rest, ice, compression, and elevation; it is depicted for you in this section. The section on REHABILITATION EXERCISES offers some exercises that can be performed after such common injuries as a sprained ankle or a shoulder injury. Even though we have stressed stretching exercises and warm-ups in earlier chapters, maintaining or developing your flexibility through warm-ups may be even more vital when you are trying to recover from an injury. We also suggest exercises for people who have tennis elbow, a hamstring injury, a groin injury, or low back pain.

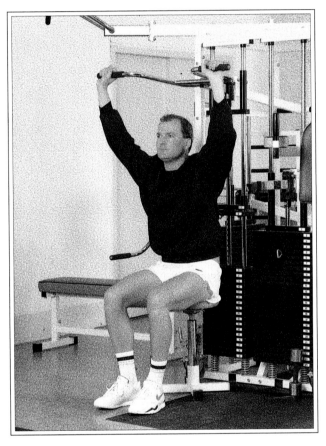

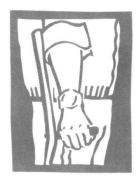

# REHABILITATION AFTER AN INJURY

RECOVERY FROM A SPORTS-RELATED injury may take several weeks, even when you act promptly and follow the recommended first-aid procedures right after the injury occurs. To speed your recovery, it is usually advisable to begin a program of rehabilitation exercises tailored to your needs – once healing has begun.

**Using an isokinetic machine**
*An isokinetic machine strengthens muscles by applying mechanical resistance to muscle groups through their range of movement. Isokinetic exercise is of great value in injury rehabilitation because you can adjust the speed, resistance, and range of the machine to meet the requirements of your injured limb.*

The most important aspect of rehabilitation is careful and controlled exercising of the damaged body part. The idea is to work out the injured joints, ligaments, or muscle tissues to the extent that their condition will allow, in order to restore them to their former healthy state.

## SEEKING HELP

The overwhelming majority of sports injuries are minor and do not require the attention of a doctor. The common-sense suggestions for treatment and rehabilitation described in THE RECOVERY PROCESS on page 122 will be enough in most cases. For obviously severe injuries or those that do not seem to heal in a reasonable period of time, a visit to a doctor is recommended.

The best person to consult if you have been injured is a doctor who treats many sports injuries. This doctor may recommend treatments such as rest, cold or heat therapy, or hydrotherapy (water treatments in a whirlpool bath or exercise pool). A set of individualized exercises, or massage, may also be recommended to restore the normal range of function to the damaged tissues. Often you are advised to begin with stretching exercises. In addition to stretching exercises, rehabilitation should include exercises to restore muscle strength, balance, coordination, and a full range of movement in the injured area. If any exercise aggravates your pain, tenderness, stiffness, or swelling, consult your doctor, who will modify your rehabilitation program accordingly. If your symptoms still persist, you may have an injury that requires additional treatment or even surgery.

If you are in traction or need a cast after an injury, ask your doctor to recommend some exercises to help maintain strength and flexibility in the parts of your body that are not immobilized.

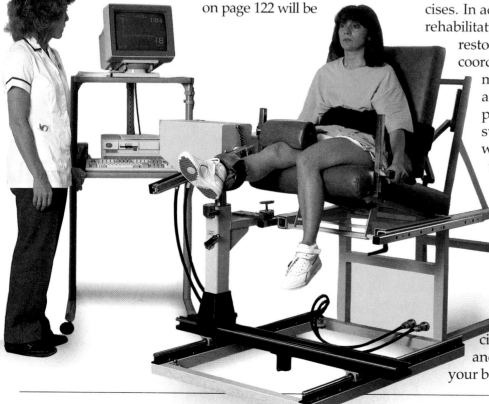

If you have a sprain or strain, your doctor may tape the affected joint for you or wrap it in an elastic bandage. If the doctor advises you to change the tape or wrap the bandage yourself before your next visit, get instructions on how to do it correctly (see also page 81).

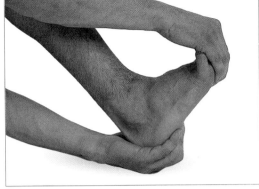

**Relieving a cramp in the foot**
*A cramp is a painful spasm in a muscle caused by excessive and prolonged contraction of the muscle fibers. To relieve a cramp in your foot, grasp your toes and gently but firmly bend them back while holding your heel with your other hand. Then knead the sole of your foot.*

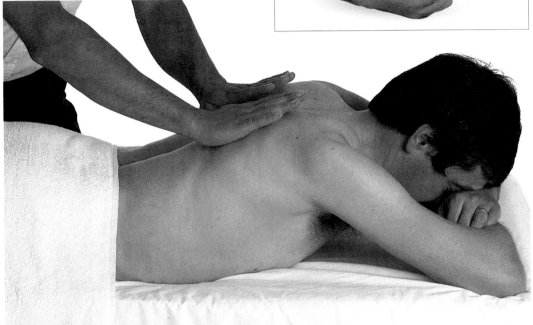

**Massage**
*Massage can reduce the pain of a muscle injury. It increases the circulation of blood and relieves pain by reducing muscle spasms. Massage also can relax you generally, increase the suppleness of your skin, and relieve stress.*

## THE HEALING PROCESS

**Reducing inflammation**
*The use of one of the nonsteroidal anti-inflammatory drugs such as aspirin, and, much less frequently, the use of oral corticosteroids or the injection of a corticosteroid drug, reduces inflammation in the area of an injury by reducing the production of prostaglandins and suppressing the release and activity of white blood cells. These medications relieve the symptoms of pain, tenderness, and swelling and help speed the healing process.*

**Before medication**

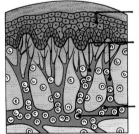

— Swelling

— Dilated blood vessels

— Increase in white blood cells

**After medication**

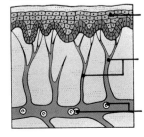

— Reduced swelling

— Blood vessels return to normal

— Fewer white blood cells

**Heated pools**
*Immersion in the warm water of a heated pool accelerates the healing of inflamed tissue and relaxes muscles and joints, making them easier to move. Moving your injured body parts in water without the full effect of gravity is also beneficial after an injury.*

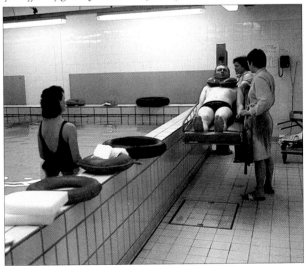

## Assisted exercise

Once a major injury, such as a fracture, has healed, you need to exercise the injured area, either by having someone move the part for you or by doing it yourself. These exercises can help reduce the stiffness in your joints and gradually restore your muscle strength.

## Medications

Minor pain following an injury may be relieved without the use of drugs by the application of ice (see THE "RICE" ROUTINE FOR FIRST AID on page 122). Minor aches and pains usually disappear eventually without drugs. If aches or pains persist, you may want to take nonsteroidal anti-inflammatory drugs (NSAIDs) such as aspirin or ibuprofen. Read the warnings on the labels of nonprescription NSAIDs. For information on the drugs you may already be taking, see A-Z OF DRUGS IN SPORTS on page 136.

## Hydrotherapy

During your recovery from a serious injury, or after an operation, your doctor may propose hydrotherapy, which involves doing exercises in a pool or bath. The water reduces the effects of gravity on your body, making the movements easier to perform.

**Hydrotherapy**
*The benefits to strained muscles and joints of immersion in warm water can be enjoyed at a health club whirlpool. However, even warm baths or showers at home can provide similar relief.*

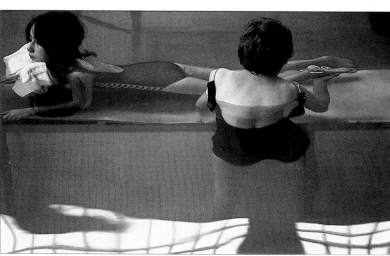

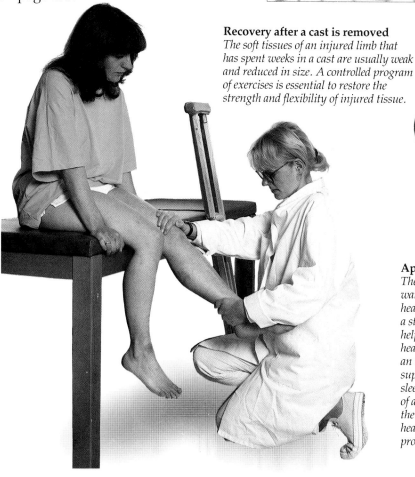

**Recovery after a cast is removed**
*The soft tissues of an injured limb that has spent weeks in a cast are usually weak and reduced in size. A controlled program of exercises is essential to restore the strength and flexibility of injured tissue.*

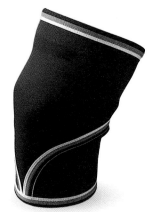

**Application of heat**
*The application of a hot-water bottle (above) or a heating pad to the area of a strained muscle can help prevent spasm. Also, heat can be kept around an injury by wearing a support such as a knee sleeve (right). Made of a synthetic material, the sleeve retains body heat and uses it to promote healing.*

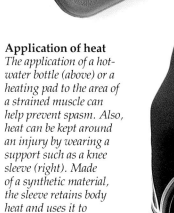

## Heat treatment

Treating an injury with heat improves the flow of blood and relaxes muscle spasms, thereby relieving pain. Heat should not be administered until at least 2 days after an injury. Started too early, heat treatment can increase bleeding and swelling, and thus aggravate an injury rather than help treat it.

# THE REHABILITATION PROGRAM

It is important that you do some gentle exercise to prevent scarring and contracting of the injured tissues. Many people avoid all activity until their pain, tenderness, and swelling have subsided – a bad decision to make. When they later try to return abruptly to their previous level of activity without appropriate rehabilitation, the injury often recurs.

## Why exercise after an injury?

Rehabilitation exercises serve three important functions. First, they improve the flexibility and strength of the damaged tissues. Next, they build up the muscles around the site of injury, which may have weakened and wasted. Finally, they help you to restore your general level of conditioning.

## Stretching exercises

After any injury, stretching exercises are invaluable for restoring full mobility and flexibility. This is because the scar tissue that remains after the injured tissue has healed tends to contract. As a result, the injured area moves awkwardly and is liable to tear again when it is forced to stretch. Stretching exercises return the injured tissue to its normal length.

## Aerobic activities

The final component of your rehabilitation program consists of aerobic activities to restore your cardiovascular fitness. Anyone who is unable to exercise for a few weeks – or even longer – inevitably becomes out of shape.

Your level of physical fitness may be restored if you resume your normal aerobic activities such as brisk walking, swimming, ice skating, or cycling.

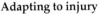

**Adapting to injury**
*Many injuries allow you to exercise other body areas fully and thereby maintain or improve your level of aerobic conditioning without compromising the healing process. For example, you can use a stationary exercise bicycle to work out while you are recovering from an injury to your arm.*

**Swimming with assistance**
*People recuperating from an injury can maintain their aerobic conditioning in the swimming pool. Devices such as a kickboard (below) allow people with an arm or leg injury to rest the injured limb while exercising.*

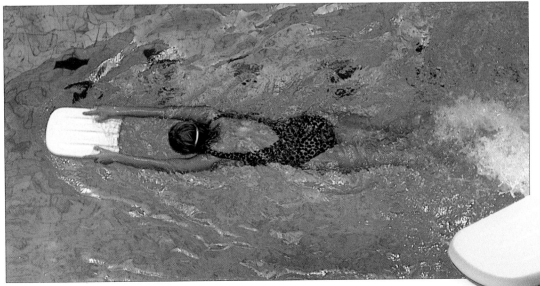

# THE RECOVERY PROCESS

Injury is a normal hazard of exercise activities and sports, but most injuries are minor and will heal quickly if you take a few steps to promote healing. However, if you ignore the symptoms and continue to exercise, you delay healing of your injury and also run a serious risk of causing more damage.

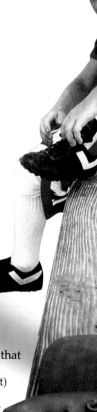

## THE "RICE" ROUTINE FOR FIRST AID

The term "RICE" is an acronym for rest, ice, compression, and elevation. These are the four basic essentials of rehabilitation for minor injuries that involve the soft tissues. RICE is usually the best immediate treatment for sprains, strains, bruises, tendinitis, and bursitis.

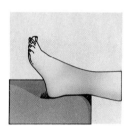

### Rest
To allow your tissues to begin healing and to reduce the amount of swelling and further bleeding in the tissues, rest the injured part of your body and avoid any unnecessary movement.

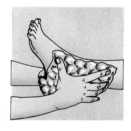

### Ice
Cold relieves pain and helps limit bruising and swelling by narrowing the blood vessels. For the first 48 hours after an injury, apply an ice pack to the injured area for 20 to 30 minutes at a time, every 3 hours.

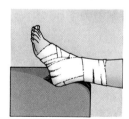

### Compression
A compression bandage worn for at least 2 days helps reduce bleeding and swelling. The bandage should cover the injured area and extend well above and below it. It should not cut off the circulation.

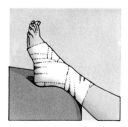

### Elevation
Raising the injured part (above the heart when possible) also helps reduce bleeding and swelling. Elevation also facilitates the draining of any fluid that has accumulated in your tissues because of the injury.

### Injury
Sports injuries may be caused by a direct blow, by overstretching muscles or tendons, or by repetitive movements of a body part. Roughly 80 percent of serious sports injuries involve soft tissues such as muscles, ligaments, tendons, or the joint lining; only about 20 percent involve a broken bone or damage to an internal organ.

### Tissue injury
A tissue injury damages blood vessels. This, in turn, results in bleeding inside the tissues, which leads to swelling around the site of the injury. As the damaged blood vessels repair themselves, a bruise may appear.

### Inflammation
Damage to tissues stimulates the release of chemicals known as prostaglandins. Along with other chemicals released inside the injured tissues, prostaglandins cause the blood vessels to enlarge and leak fluid, which results in the familiar features of inflammation – redness, warmth, swelling, and tenderness.

### Pain
The skin and soft tissues contain many specialized nerve endings that feel pain when a nearby area is damaged. "RICE" (see above left) helps relieve pain, and a non-steroidal anti-inflammatory drug (NSAID) may be prescribed to reduce pain and swelling.

## APPLYING HEAT

You can apply heat to the injured area to aid healing after the first 48 hours (or once the swelling around the injury has been controlled as much as possible). In general, do not apply heat to an area that continues to swell.

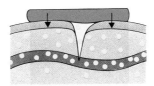
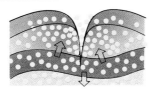
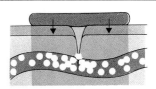

**1** Fluid leaks from the blood vessels around the injury and accumulates in the tissues. The bleeding and tissue damage cause more inflammation.

**2** Ice packs applied soon after the injury contract the damaged blood vessels, which reduces bleeding. Ice also reduces swelling and inflammation.

**3** When the swelling stops, heat can be applied to dilate (widen) the blood vessels, which allows blood cells needed for healing to reach the injured area.

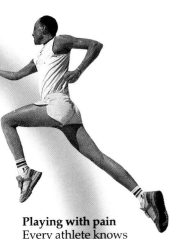

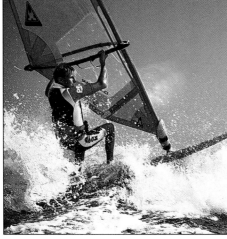

**Exercise**
As healing continues, scar tissue may develop to replace the tissues that were injured. This new tissue is shorter and more rigid than the original tissue, so it is easily damaged. You should begin stretching and strengthening exercises (see page 124) gently and gradually to bring back the full range of flexibility to the injured area.

**Playing with pain**
Every athlete knows that it is possible, in the short term, to ignore the pain and other symptoms of an injury. But doing this can lead to further injury, repeating the cycle of pain and inflammation.

**Healing**
Once the healing process is complete, the injured area should be back almost to full strength and flexibility. Occasionally, a severe injury or repeated injuries to the same area lead to a slight weakness in that area.

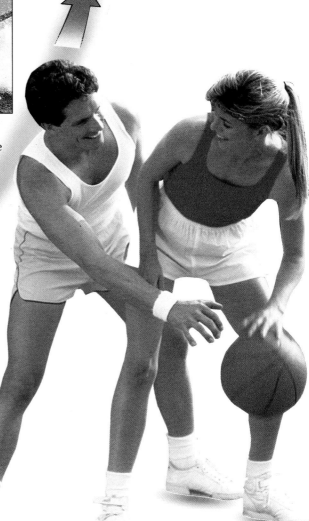

**First aid**
Following an injury, you should stop exercising immediately and rest the injured body part. Begin treatment (see THE "RICE" ROUTINE FOR FIRST AID, far left) as soon as possible, and do not start exercising again until both the pain and the inflammation have stopped.

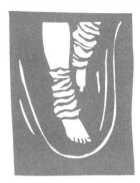

# REHABILITATION EXERCISES

As is true of any exercise program, rehabilitation exercises are valuable to the extent that you are disciplined and persist in them throughout your period of disability. Rehabilitation exercises should include a stretching sequence as well as movements designed to restore strength, balance, coordination, and a full range of movement to the injured tissues.

If you injure a muscle, tendon, or ligament, you can safely do some gentle exercises as soon as the pain and swelling subside and you are able to move the injured part without aggravating the pain. This may be some time after the first 48 hours. Supervised exercise to uninjured body parts helps maintain your overall strength and flexibility while the injured part heals.

If you have broken a bone, your doctor will probably immobilize it in a cast for several weeks to allow complete healing. The cast almost always covers the joint above and below the fracture site. When the cast comes off, you may begin a rehabilitation program to restore strength and flexibility to the muscles, tendons, and joints weakened and stiffened by the prolonged immobilization.

## PACING YOURSELF

At the beginning of your rehabilitation program, do not perform any exercise that increases your pain. You may be able to do only a few mild exercises for a short period of time at first, but gradually you will be able to increase your range of motion. Work through each exercise slowly, stopping and resting for a while if the injured area becomes painful. Try to do three sessions a day and build up to doing 10 repetitions of each exercise. It may take several weeks to increase the number of exercises you can perform and the time you spend on them. You may feel sore between exercise sessions. Remember that overexerting yourself too soon does more harm than good.

**Leg lifts aid recovery**
*If your leg has been immobilized after an injury, you will experience weakness and stiffness in the limb from lack of use. Performing the side leg lift (below) helps to strengthen the abductor muscles, which run from the hip to the knee on the outside of your leg.*

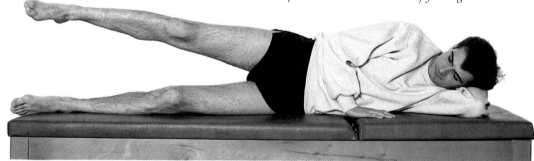

**WARNING**
When you can successfully do all the exercises in your recovery program, you may be ready to return to your preinjury exercises or sports. If you start training or competing before you recover, you run the great risk of aggravating the injury. If you are unable to make progress in your exercise program because of persistent pain, tenderness, stiffness, or swelling, consult your doctor. You may have an injury that requires additional treatment.

# EXERCISES AFTER AN ANKLE SPRAIN

The goal of rehabilitation exercises for the ankle is to restore the full range of movement and balance provided by this joint. Unless your balance is fully restored, the risk of reinjury is extremely high.

## Stretching exercises

**1** Lie flat on the floor and move your feet forward and backward, keeping both of your heels in contact with the floor.

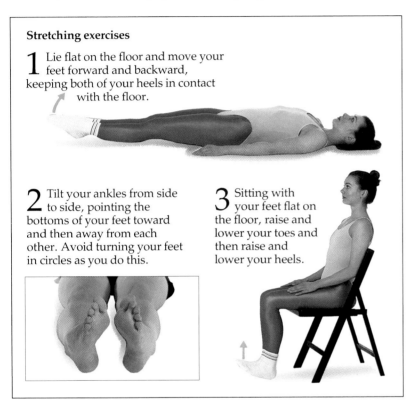

**2** Tilt your ankles from side to side, pointing the bottoms of your feet toward and then away from each other. Avoid turning your feet in circles as you do this.

**3** Sitting with your feet flat on the floor, raise and lower your toes and then raise and lower your heels.

## Exercises to improve balance and coordination

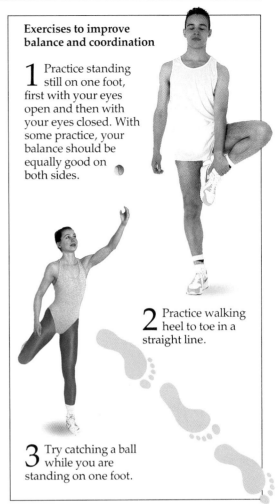

**1** Practice standing still on one foot, first with your eyes open and then with your eyes closed. With some practice, your balance should be equally good on both sides.

**2** Practice walking heel to toe in a straight line.

**3** Try catching a ball while you are standing on one foot.

## Strengthening exercises

**1** Put one foot on top of the other and pull up with the lower foot while pushing down with the upper foot. Press your feet together for a few seconds. Repeat with the other foot.

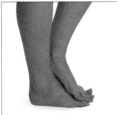

**2** Press the inside edges of your feet together, then cross your feet and press the outside edges together.

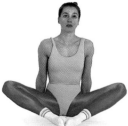
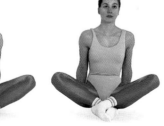

**3** (Not shown.) Stand on your toes, then alternately on your heels. Walk on your toes and then on your heels.

**4** Walk and jump sideways to your right, then to your left.

**5** Secure a 1-pound weight to your foot and move the foot upward and outward.

**6** Hop forward, then to the side, on each foot.

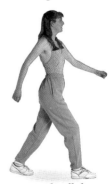

**7** Walk briskly, building up your speed and distance over several days. You can also try walking or running backward.

**8** Once you can do all these exercises without pain or difficulty, start kicking a ball against a wall using first the top of your foot, then the outside edge, and finally your instep.

## EXERCISES FOR TENNIS ELBOW

It is important to exercise not only your arm but also common sense in trying these movements to help rehabilitate your forearm muscles. To reduce the chance of a recurrence of the elbow injury, stop if you feel any pain or discomfort.

### Strength and mobility exercises

**1** Rest your injured forearm flat on a table with your hand hanging over the edge. Move your wrist slowly up and then down, holding it in each position for a few seconds.

**2** (Not shown.) Repeat the wrist movements described above, slowly and then more rapidly, holding a small weight in your hand.

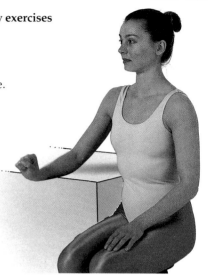

### Stretching exercises

Start stretching the muscles on the back of your forearm by bending the wrist and fingers of your uninjured arm downward, while you keep your sore elbow slightly bent. You will feel a slight pull in the forearm muscles; hold this pose for a few seconds each time.

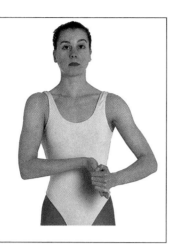

**3** Bend and straighten your elbow, then rotate your forearm up and down, so that the palm of your hand faces up and then down. Repeat each of these exercises while holding a small weight in your hand.

**4** Try to perform some push-ups; stop immediately if you feel any pain.

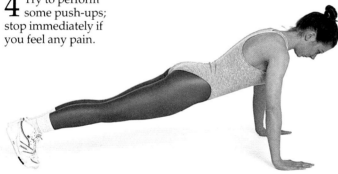

**5** Put a thick rubber band around your fingertips. Spread and then relax your fingers to stretch and release the band.

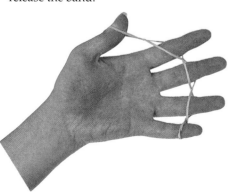

**6** Once you can do exercises 1 through 5 without experiencing pain on the outside of your elbow or in your forearm, practice screwing and unscrewing movements with a screwdriver. Choose a screwdriver with a long handle to reduce the stress placed on your forearm muscles.

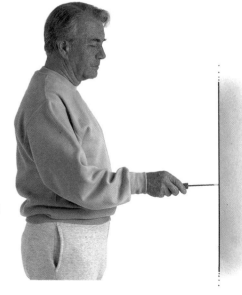

**7** Once you have worked through this program of exercises, you may carefully start throwing a ball and using a tennis racket again.

# CASE HISTORY
## PAINFUL ELBOW

FRANK PLAYS TENNIS AT LEAST **two or three times a week. He first noticed discomfort in his elbow a couple of days ago. Since then the pain has gotten steadily worse and has now spread down his forearm, making it impossible for him to play tennis and difficult to lift or carry anything. He also feels pain when he shakes hands or opens doors.**

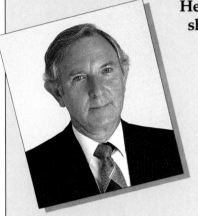

### PERSONAL DETAILS
**Name** Frank Jackson
**Age** 58
**Occupation** Economist
**Family** Both Frank's parents died in their 70s, his father of pneumonia and his mother of a stroke.

### MEDICAL BACKGROUND
Frank rarely sees his doctor. His last office visit was about 3 years ago, after he sprained his ankle.

### THE CONSULTATION
Frank describes the pain in his elbow and forearm to his doctor. His doctor asks him what he has been doing recently that could have brought on this pain. Frank replies that he doesn't remember hitting his elbow against anything but that it feels as if he has bruised it. Frank says that recently he has been playing a lot of tennis and wonders if he has overexerted himself. Over the past few weeks he has been playing tennis virtually every day.

The doctor examines Frank carefully and finds a tender spot over the bony area on the outside of Frank's right elbow. The pain in his elbow and forearm becomes much worse when the doctor gently but firmly pushes his hand against the hand of Frank's injured arm.

### THE DIAGNOSIS
The doctor tells Frank that he has an injury that is commonly called TENNIS ELBOW. Tennis elbow is a condition in which the tendons on the outside of the elbow become inflamed, resulting in pain, some swelling, and tenderness. It is caused by repeatedly hitting backhand shots using the wrist instead of the whole arm, or by twisting the forearm while gripping tightly. Tennis elbow is common in people who play a lot of tennis or other racket

**A telltale pain**
*Frank's injury makes it painful for him to push against his doctor's outstretched hand. By doing so, he contracts the muscles and puts stress on the tendons, causing his symptoms.*

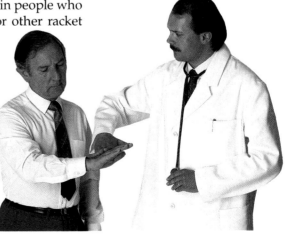

sports, especially those who are using a racket with the wrong size grip for them. Despite its name, tennis elbow can develop after any activity that overworks the muscles on the back of the forearm. These muscles bend your wrist and fingers upward. The tendons that join these muscles to the elbow become inflamed when the muscles are overworked.

### THE TREATMENT
Frank's doctor recommends that he rest his arm for a few days until gripping and lifting no longer produce pain. He is also told to apply ice for 20 to 30 minutes every 3 hours throughout the day. The doctor suggests that Frank try the RICE routine of rest, ice, compression, and elevation (see page 122).

### THE OUTLOOK
Frank returns to his doctor a week later with only slight discomfort in his elbow when he grips or lifts something. The doctor recommends some exercises to help Frank regain strength and flexibility in his arm and to reduce the risk of reinjury. He also suggests that Frank check the size of the grip on his racket and that he consider taking lessons to improve his technique.

# EXERCISES FOR AN INJURED SHOULDER

Once the initial pain and swelling of a shoulder injury have passed, you can begin gentle stretching and strengthening exercises for the different muscles. (Swimming may also help, but be careful not to do too much too early and don't do any stroke that feels uncomfortable.) Stop doing any of the following exercises immediately if you feel pain or discomfort in your injured shoulder.

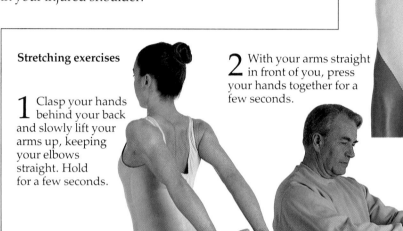

## Stretching exercises

**1** Clasp your hands behind your back and slowly lift your arms up, keeping your elbows straight. Hold for a few seconds.

**2** With your arms straight in front of you, press your hands together for a few seconds.

**3** Bend the arm attached to the affected shoulder over your head, pull your wrist with the other hand, and bend your body gently in the same direction in which you are pulling.

**4** Raise your arms straight up above your head and reach backward slowly.

## Mobility exercises

**1** Lie flat and move your arms away from your sides; first move them up in front of you and then above your head.

**2** Lie flat and put your hands behind your head, elbows bent; move your elbows up and down.

**3** Stand with the hand on your "good" side resting on a chair, lean forward, and gently try to swing the arm attached to your injured shoulder forward, backward, and sideways, and then in circles of increasing size.

**4** Stand with your arms by your sides; cautiously swing your arms forward and backward, bringing your hands together in front of you and behind you.

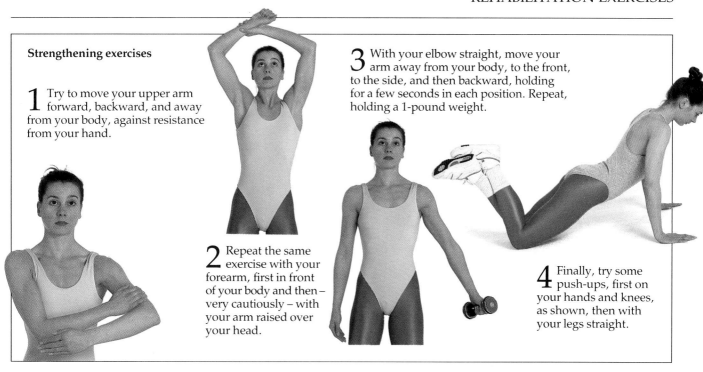

### Strengthening exercises

**1** Try to move your upper arm forward, backward, and away from your body, against resistance from your hand.

**2** Repeat the same exercise with your forearm, first in front of your body and then – very cautiously – with your arm raised over your head.

**3** With your elbow straight, move your arm away from your body, to the front, to the side, and then backward, holding for a few seconds in each position. Repeat, holding a 1-pound weight.

**4** Finally, try some push-ups, first on your hands and knees, as shown, then with your legs straight.

## EXERCISES AFTER A KNEE INJURY

After any injury to your knee it is important to start doing exercises promptly to maintain the strength in the quadriceps muscles, which are located at the front of your thigh. Once the injury starts to heal and the pain and swelling subside, you can add some exercises that involve bending your knee.

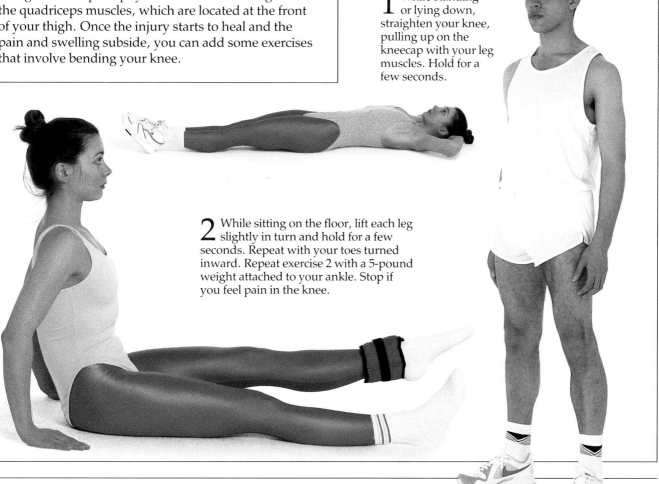

### Quadriceps exercises

**1** While standing or lying down, straighten your knee, pulling up on the kneecap with your leg muscles. Hold for a few seconds.

**2** While sitting on the floor, lift each leg slightly in turn and hold for a few seconds. Repeat with your toes turned inward. Repeat exercise 2 with a 5-pound weight attached to your ankle. Stop if you feel pain in the knee.

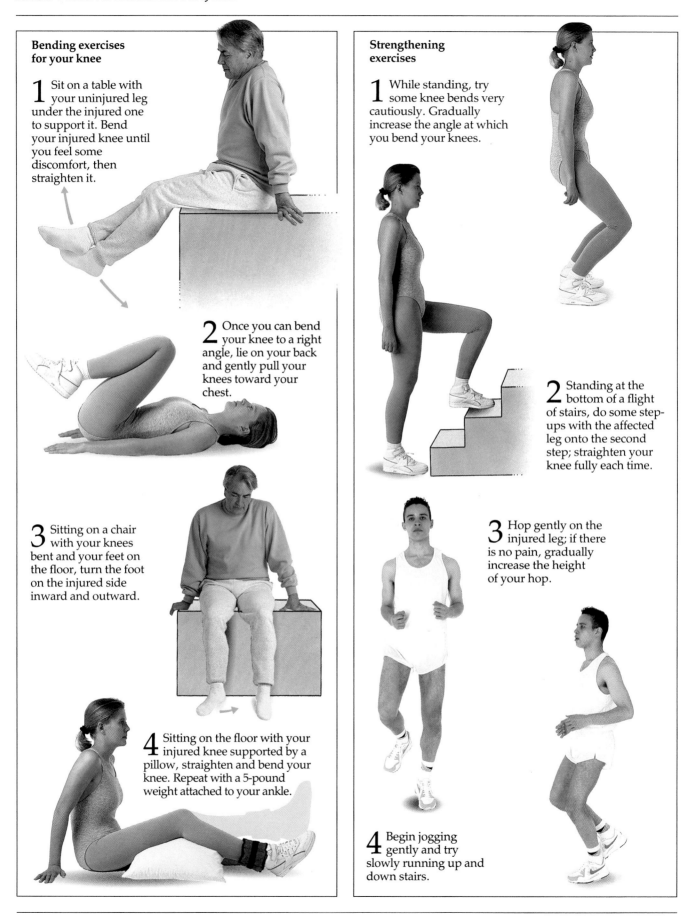

**Bending exercises for your knee**

**1** Sit on a table with your uninjured leg under the injured one to support it. Bend your injured knee until you feel some discomfort, then straighten it.

**2** Once you can bend your knee to a right angle, lie on your back and gently pull your knees toward your chest.

**3** Sitting on a chair with your knees bent and your feet on the floor, turn the foot on the injured side inward and outward.

**4** Sitting on the floor with your injured knee supported by a pillow, straighten and bend your knee. Repeat with a 5-pound weight attached to your ankle.

**Strengthening exercises**

**1** While standing, try some knee bends very cautiously. Gradually increase the angle at which you bend your knees.

**2** Standing at the bottom of a flight of stairs, do some step-ups with the affected leg onto the second step; straighten your knee fully each time.

**3** Hop gently on the injured leg; if there is no pain, gradually increase the height of your hop.

**4** Begin jogging gently and try slowly running up and down stairs.

# EXERCISES FOR BACK PAIN

As your back pain eases, you should be able to do some gentle exercises.
Once you can do all these exercises without discomfort, you can resume your
normal activities. Be especially cautious about doing any exercise that causes
pain; stop immediately if your back hurts.

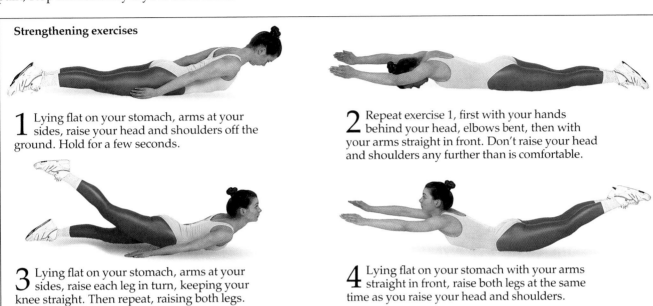

**Strengthening exercises**

1 Lying flat on your stomach, arms at your
sides, raise your head and shoulders off the
ground. Hold for a few seconds.

2 Repeat exercise 1, first with your hands
behind your head, elbows bent, then with
your arms straight in front. Don't raise your head
and shoulders any further than is comfortable.

3 Lying flat on your stomach, arms at your
sides, raise each leg in turn, keeping your
knee straight. Then repeat, raising both legs.

4 Lying flat on your stomach with your arms
straight in front, raise both legs at the same
time as you raise your head and shoulders.

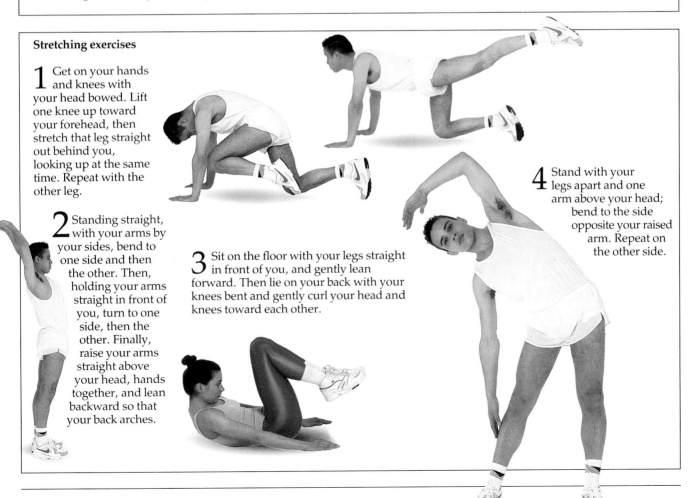

**Stretching exercises**

1 Get on your hands
and knees with
your head bowed. Lift
one knee up toward
your forehead, then
stretch that leg straight
out behind you,
looking up at the same
time. Repeat with the
other leg.

2 Standing straight,
with your arms by
your sides, bend to
one side and then
the other. Then,
holding your arms
straight in front of
you, turn to one
side, then the
other. Finally,
raise your arms
straight above
your head, hands
together, and lean
backward so that
your back arches.

3 Sit on the floor with your legs straight
in front of you, and gently lean
forward. Then lie on your back with your
knees bent and gently curl your head and
knees toward each other.

4 Stand with your
legs apart and one
arm above your head;
bend to the side
opposite your raised
arm. Repeat on
the other side.

**Mobility exercises
for your back**

1 Get on your hands and knees and arch your back upward while bending your head down. Then arch your back downward with your head up.

2 Lie on your back with your knees bent and your feet flat on the floor; keeping your knees together, rock them from left to right. With your knees still bent, push your lower back down onto the floor, then arch it away from the floor. Finally, raise both your back and your buttocks off the floor.

3 Lie on your back with your legs straight. Then very carefully raise one leg up toward your waist from the hip while hugging the floor with your other leg as much as possible. Repeat with the other side.

4 Lie on your back with your arms out to the side at right angles. Lift one leg straight up in the air, then swing it across the other leg, keeping your shoulders on the floor. Repeat with the other leg.

5 Lie on your back with your arms out at right angles to your body, and move your right foot up so that it rests on the inside of your left knee. Then slowly turn your back to the left so that your bent knee moves toward the floor, keeping your shoulders on the floor. Repeat on the other side.

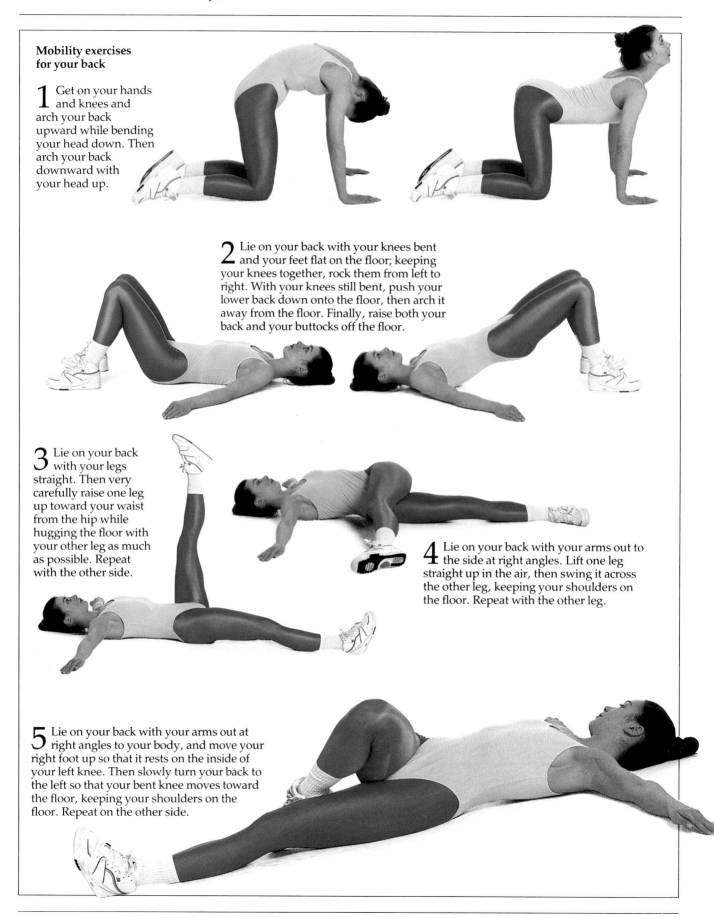

# CASE HISTORY
# PAIN IN THE BACK AND LEGS

**E**RIC HAS ALWAYS BEEN an avid golfer. Over the past few months he has been practicing nonstop for the annual state championships. He has also been doing a series of exercises to help him get into top form. One week before the competition, following a vigorous 18 holes, Eric awoke with severe pain in the lower part of his back. The pain spread into his left buttock and down the back of his left leg. Eric called an orthopedist that day.

### PERSONAL DETAILS
**Name** Eric T. Wilson
**Age** 54
**Occupation** Librarian
**Family** Eric's mother is in excellent health. His father has Parkinson's disease but is still able to care for himself and go for walks.

## THE CONSULTATION
Eric describes his pain and tells his doctor that he is unable to stand up straight. His left leg feels weak and he has numbness and tingling in his left foot. While examining Eric, the doctor finds a muscle spasm on the left side of his lumbar spine (the middle portion of the spine). The spasm is causing Eric to lean to the left. When he lies flat on the examination table, Eric is able to raise his right leg to an angle of 80 degrees. His left leg, however, can be lifted to an angle of only 20 degrees. Performing this movement aggravates the pain in both his back and his leg. Eric has an area of tenderness between the lowest vertebra in the lumbar region of the spine and the top of the sacrum. The doctor arranges for Eric to have X-rays taken of his lumbar spine.

## THE DIAGNOSIS
After looking at Eric's X-rays, the doctor says that his symptoms are probably caused by a PROLAPSED (RUPTURED) DISC in the lower part of his back. A fragment of the disc is placing pressure on one of the left lumbar nerve roots at the point where it emerges from the spine. This pressure is causing the pain in Eric's back and left leg and the numbness, tingling, and weakness in his left foot. The doctor tests Eric's reflexes by tapping his knees and ankles with a small hammer; when he tests Eric's left ankle, he finds that the ankle does not react as it naturally should – indicating that the disc is interfering with the functioning of the sciatic nerve.

## THE TREATMENT
Eric is advised to rest at home on a flat surface with a pillow under his knees to reduce the stress on the lower part of his spine. To relieve the spasm in his back, the doctor prescribes painkillers containing codeine and a nonsteroidal anti-inflammatory drug. The doctor also recommends that he apply heat to the painful area in the form of a heating pad for several days.

A week later, the pain and stiffness in the lower part of Eric's back are alleviated somewhat, but he is still having some twinges of pain in his left leg. After the doctor is satisfied that Eric has sufficiently recovered to begin rehabilitation exercises, the doctor shows him how to stretch and strengthen his back and also the abdominal muscles that support the back. He also advises Eric to lose about 10 pounds to help reduce the strain on the lower part of his back.

## THE OUTLOOK
Within 2 weeks, Eric is free of pain and has regained a full range of movement in his spine. After reviewing Eric's account of his frequent games of golf, the doctor advises him against injuring himself again through overuse. He suggests that Eric exercise moderation and cut down on the number of times per week that he plays golf.

**Muscle spasm**
*The muscles on the left side of Eric's spine had gone into spasm, making it difficult and painful for him to stand upright.*

# EXERCISES AFTER A GROIN INJURY

For the first few days after a groin injury or after hernia repair surgery, walking at even a slow pace will be uncomfortable. However, try to stand up and walk as straight as the pain allows. Slowly increase the amount of walking you do, and gradually start to do the following stretching and strengthening exercises. Once you can perform these exercises without feeling discomfort, you should be ready to return to normal activities. Swimming and walking are good forms of exercise at this stage. It is important, however, to avoid any heavy lifting or vigorous stretching for at least the first 3 months after a hernia operation.

**Abdomen-strengthening exercises**

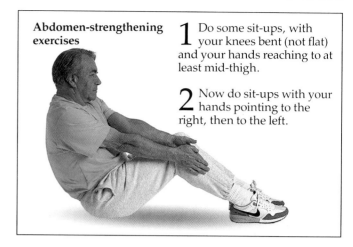

**1** Do some sit-ups, with your knees bent (not flat) and your hands reaching to at least mid-thigh.

**2** Now do sit-ups with your hands pointing to the right, then to the left.

## Abdominal exercises

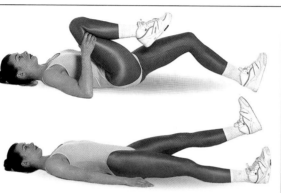

**1** Lie on your back and bend your right knee toward your chest, with your left knee held slightly bent. Then repeat the exercise, bending your left knee toward your chest.

**2** Lie on your back and slowly raise each leg in turn a few inches off the floor. Try to keep your knee straight.

## Groin-strengthening exercises

**1** (Not shown.) Lie on your back, with your legs straight; press your feet and knees together for a few seconds at a time.

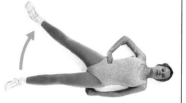

**2** Lie flat on your back and, keeping your right leg straight, move it carefully as far away as possible from your other leg, then bring it back again. Repeat the exercise, moving your left leg.

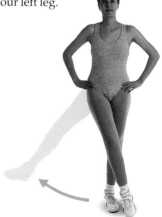

**3** Once you can do exercise 2, gently do it from a standing position, crossing your moving leg over the stationary one each time you swing it back.

## Muscle stretches

**1** Lie face down and raise each leg in turn off the floor until you feel a pull in the top of your thigh. Hold for a count of five. Do not jerk or bounce the movement.

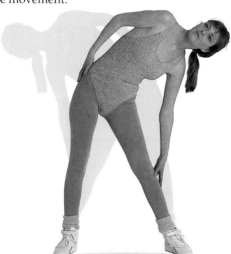

**2** (Not shown.) Lie on your back, knees bent and feet together, and slowly move your knees apart until you feel a pull on the inside of your thighs. Hold for a count of five. Be careful not to jerk or bounce while doing this exercise.

**3** Stand with your legs wide apart and lean your torso slowly to the right until you feel a pull in your left groin. Then repeat the exercise, this time leaning to the left.

## EXERCISES AFTER A HAMSTRING INJURY

For the first few days after a hamstring injury you will feel pain and tenderness at the back of your thigh. You may also find that you walk with a limp because it is painful to straighten your injured leg. After 48 hours' rest you should carefully start to perform some gentle stretching exercises. Try to straighten your leg as much as the pain allows when you stand or walk, and slowly increase the amount of walking that you do.

**Hamstring stretches**

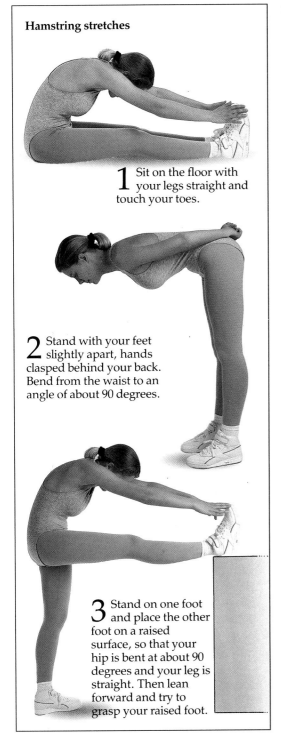

1 Sit on the floor with your legs straight and touch your toes.

2 Stand with your feet slightly apart, hands clasped behind your back. Bend from the waist to an angle of about 90 degrees.

3 Stand on one foot and place the other foot on a raised surface, so that your hip is bent at about 90 degrees and your leg is straight. Then lean forward and try to grasp your raised foot.

**Hamstring-strengthening exercises**

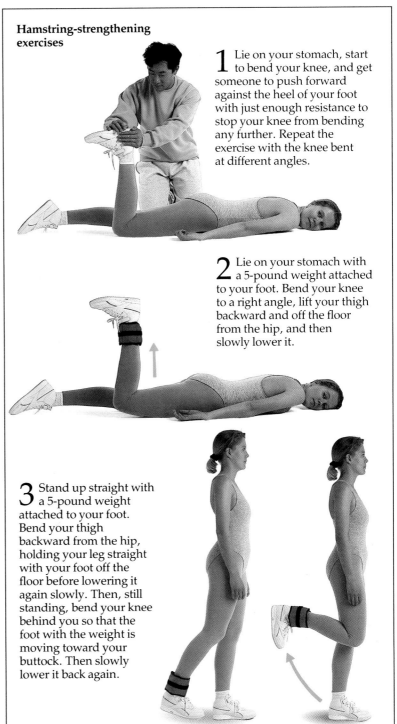

1 Lie on your stomach, start to bend your knee, and get someone to push forward against the heel of your foot with just enough resistance to stop your knee from bending any further. Repeat the exercise with the knee bent at different angles.

2 Lie on your stomach with a 5-pound weight attached to your foot. Bend your knee to a right angle, lift your thigh backward and off the floor from the hip, and then slowly lower it.

3 Stand up straight with a 5-pound weight attached to your foot. Bend your thigh backward from the hip, holding your leg straight with your foot off the floor before lowering it again slowly. Then, still standing, bend your knee behind you so that the foot with the weight is moving toward your buttock. Then slowly lower it back again.

# A-Z OF DRUGS IN SPORTS

Many adults take at least one drug every day. The most common drugs used in the US are alcohol, caffeine, and nicotine. However, people also make periodic or regular use of a wide range of medications (over-the-counter and prescription preparations alike) to relieve their medical conditions. Some people abuse substances such as anabolic steroids, which they hope will enhance their conditioning or their performance in sports.

In this section, we discuss drugs and how they might affect your physical fitness or performance. Many common remedies for colds, coughs, hay fever, and diarrhea contain low doses of substances that allegedly improve performance; however, very few of them actually have any impact on performance. Also, sports authorities have banned the use of many drugs by those competing in organized athletic competitions.

## ALCOHOL

Drinking alcohol has no place in exercise or sports. Some people imagine that drinking a small amount of alcohol before exercising may help them relax or may be effective in reducing a tremor. Others think there are benefits from smoking marijuana, an illegal narcotic. However, using these drugs during a workout causes loss of coordination and a delay in reaction time.

In addition, alcohol increases the risk of hypothermia (a dangerous drop in body temperature) when you exercise in cold weather because it creates a false sense of warmth by dilating (widening) the blood vessels under your skin. This results in an increase in blood flow that makes your skin feel warm; however, heat loss from your body increases.

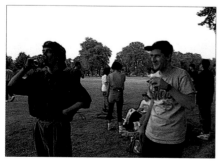

**Alcohol before exercise**
*Drinking alcoholic beverages before exercise increases your loss of body heat; also, it impairs your coordination, reaction time, and ability to make quick decisions.*

## AMPHETAMINES

Amphetamines are stimulants that were once widely prescribed as dieting medications because of their ability to reduce appetite. Amphetamines are commonly abused because they also can improve your mood and inhibit fatigue. In high doses they may cause altered perception and hallucinations.

The use of amphetamines is prohibited in all competitive sports. Proponents claim that amphetamines enhance performance by minimizing or masking the effects of fatigue and by increasing aggression, but controlled studies do not show any benefit to performance. Use of these drugs can result in a number of dangerous side effects. These include collapse from overheating, an excessive increase in blood pressure, episodes of irregular heartbeat, and seizures. Amphetamines are also highly addictive.

## ANTIBIOTICS

Antibiotics are prescription drugs that treat infections caused by bacteria. Antibiotics occasionally impair your performance by causing symptoms such as nausea and diarrhea. However, exercising with a major infection should be avoided in any event, since you may increase the risk of complications.

## ANTIHISTAMINES

Antihistamines relieve the symptoms of any allergic reaction, including allergic rhinitis (hay fever), hives, and swelling caused by insect bites or stings. If you are taking antihistamines and plan to engage in vigorous exercise, you should be aware that some of these drugs commonly cause drowsiness and dizziness; some people may experience blurred vision after taking antihistamines. Drugs that contain chlorpheniramine or diphenhydramine may impair your athletic performance.

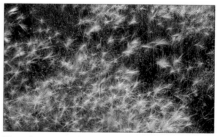

**Hay-fever medications**
*Many people are allergic to pollen from trees, grass, and weeds – such as goldenrod – and thus require medication when the pollen count is high.*

## ANTI-INFLAMMATORY DRUGS

Nonsteroidal anti-inflammatory drugs (NSAIDs) are used to relieve the symptoms of arthritis, including pain, stiffness, and swelling, and also to relieve pain caused by injury to a ligament, muscle, or tendon. NSAIDs have also been shown to accelerate recovery. Some commonly used NSAIDs are aspirin, ibuprofen, indomethacin, naproxen, piroxicam, and sulindac. You should never take NSAIDs to relieve pain during exercise because you could aggravate the injury and cause permanent damage to the affected area.

## ASTHMA DRUGS

Drugs that are prescribed to prevent or relieve asthma improve the flow of air to and from the lungs. Commonly used drugs include inhaled cromolyn sodium, corticosteroid drugs, and bronchodilators. If you hope to participate in competitive sports, make sure your asthma medication does not include any prohibited stimulants such as isoproterenol, ephedrine, or phenylephrine; if it does, consult your doctor. See also the information on asthma in SHOULD I EXERCISE IF I HAVE OTHER DISORDERS? on page 53.

## BETA BLOCKERS

Beta blockers are drugs prescribed to treat angina pectoris, cardiac arrhythmia (an irregular heartbeat), or high blood pressure. They are also effective in prevention of migraine headaches and relief of symptoms of anxiety such as shaking, palpitations, and sweating. However, beta blockers impair aerobic exercise performance. Ask your doctor about appropriate exercise for you if you are taking beta blockers.

## BLOOD DOPING

In blood doping, a potentially dangerous prohibited procedure in competitive sports, a pint of blood is removed from the athlete and stored in a blood bank. The athlete's blood volume and the number of red blood cells in the circulation are then naturally and rapidly replenished. Just before an important competition, the athlete's blood is re-infused, increasing the concentration of hemoglobin, the red blood cell pigment. A new variation is the use of the drug erythropoietin, which stimulates the body to make more blood.

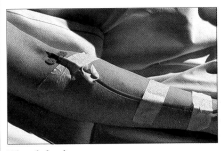

**Blood doping**
*The extraction and reinfusion of blood cells is sometimes abused in an attempt to improve the delivery of oxygen to the muscles.*

## CAFFEINE

Caffeine is a stimulant found in coffee, tea, and cola drinks. Caffeine is also included in some cold remedies and painkillers and is available in tablet form over-the-counter as a nonprescription drug.

Caffeine has a number of effects on the body. It reduces drowsiness and fatigue and may speed up your reaction time. It stimulates your heart to beat faster and more strongly and also improves energy production in the muscles, enhancing your performance during exercise.

However, in high doses, caffeine may cause palpitations, headache, abdominal pain, nausea, vomiting, restlessness, nervousness, and a tremor. Although caffeine is on the list of prohibited stimulants for athletic competition, an athlete is disqualified only when caffeine is found in large amounts in a urine sample.

## COCAINE

Cocaine is an illegal and highly addictive stimulant drug. Athletes who use it are prohibited from all organized competition. Although cocaine may enhance performance by improving mood and reducing the perception of pain, it can also cause a number of dangerous side effects, including an irregular heartbeat, negative changes in personality, and damage to the lining of the nose from regular inhalation. High doses of cocaine may cause seizures or precipitate an episode of psychosis, a form of mental illness. Cocaine can also result in death, even for a first-time user.

## COLD AND COUGH REMEDIES

Many people take tablets, capsules, nasal sprays, or cough medicines for relief of symptoms of the common cold. These preparations contain an analgesic (painkiller) and may also contain decongestants or ANTIHISTAMINES (see page 136), which are stimulants prohibited by most sports authorities. You should avoid any preparation that contains ephedrine, pseudoephedrine, phenylephrine, or phenylpropanolamine for at least 12 hours before athletic competition. You should also avoid any cough syrup that contains codeine. Codeine is prohibited in organized sports, even when you ingest it in tiny amounts as a cough suppressant. The casual exerciser needs to know that codeine may cause drowsiness or dizziness, especially if you take it with alcohol (which is also contained in many cough syrups).

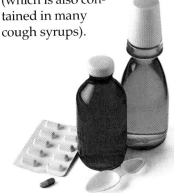

**Over-the-counter remedies**
*Many cough and cold remedies contain substances that could negatively affect your performance.*

137

## CORTICOSTEROID INJECTIONS

An injection of a corticosteroid drug, which produces reactions similar to those induced by natural corticosteroid hormones in the body, may be administered by a doctor to treat an inflamed tendon, ligament, joint, or bone surface that has not responded to conservative treatment. Corticosteroids are used to treat inflammation that does not respond to anti-inflammatory drugs. The corticosteroid is usually given with a local anesthetic. Once the anesthetic has worn off, there may be an increase in pain for the next day or so.

Doctors usually suggest resting the inflamed area completely for the first 2 days; then you may gradually start exercising again.

## DIARRHEA REMEDIES

Loperamide, codeine, or diphenoxylate with atropine are sometimes suggested for attacks of acute diarrhea, such as those that occur after ingesting contaminated food or water. Possible side effects of these drugs include nausea and vomiting, either of which will make it uncomfortable for you to exercise.

You should avoid taking any anti-diarrheal medicine that contains codeine within 12 hours of any athletic competition, because even small amounts of codeine are prohibited in those who are in competition. As a substitute, use a prepared electrolyte solution or an oral rehydration solution (water, sugar, and salt) as part of a fluid-only diet until the diarrhea is alleviated.

## DIETING MEDICATIONS

Most nonprescription medications for weight loss contain a prohibited stimulant (see also CAFFEINE on page 137 and DIURETICS on this page). Most doctors advise against taking diet pills in any case.

## DIURETICS

Diuretics are used as a treatment for heart failure and high blood pressure. They are prohibited in organized athletics because some athletes take them to flush out traces of other banned substances, such as narcotics, stimulants, or anabolic steroids, from the body. Diuretics have also been abused in the past in boxing, wrestling, or judo by competitors who have gained weight and who are now trying to reduce and "make the weight" through water loss. Using a diuretic to lose weight is dangerous for any person, but especially for athletes because there usually is not enough time between the weigh-in and the competition to replace the lost body fluids and salts. As a result, there is a high risk that fatigue, muscle weakness, and dehydration will impair performance during exertion.

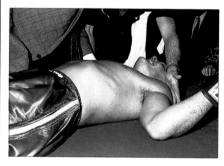

**Diuretic abuse**
*Boxers may have fatigue, muscle weakness, and dehydration if they abuse diuretics to help them reach their weight classification.*

## HAY-FEVER REMEDIES

If you have allergic rhinitis, or hay fever, and plan to take part in organized athletics, do not use a decongestant or nasal preparation that contains the prohibited stimulants ephedrine, pseudoephedrine, phenylephrine, or phenylpropanolamine. Acceptable alternative treatments for rhinitis include ear or nose drops or sprays containing cromolyn sodium, and nasal sprays that contain a corticosteroid drug.

## HORMONES

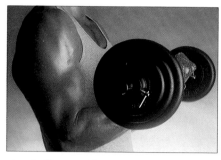

**Anabolic steroids**
*Some weight lifters abuse steroids to enhance their strength and appearance. This practice carries serious risks to health.*

Most sports authorities prohibit the use of all bodybuilding hormones, including anabolic steroids, which are probably most often abused to improve performance. Anabolic steroids consist of a group of substances that produce an effect similar to that of the male sex hormone testosterone. Athletes take them to increase muscle development by increasing production of muscle protein. Training harder stimulates protein production, which leads to an increase in muscle bulk and strength. Anabolic steroids carry risks of liver damage, liver tumors, injury to the adrenal glands, and impotence in men.

Synthetic growth hormone is also abused to build up muscles. In nature, the hormone is produced by the pituitary gland (a small gland at the base of the brain) and released in large quantities during childhood and adolescence to promote normal growth. Synthetic growth hormone is sometimes prescribed for children who are not growing because they produce abnormally low levels of growth hormone.

Adults who abuse synthetic growth hormone to increase muscle strength often find that it causes muscle weakness. This hormone may also cause coarsening of the skin and may cause the voice to deepen. Prolonged use may cause high blood pressure.

## LINIMENTS

Liniments are ointments or creams that you rub onto an area of skin to relieve pain and stiffness in the underlying tissues. Some liniments contain chemicals that relieve bruising or inflammation. Others contain rubefacients, substances that increase blood flow through the skin, causing a feeling of heat.

The application of a liniment may make a painful area feel better temporarily by acting as a counterirritant on the pain receptors in the skin. However, there is no evidence that liniment has any major effect below the skin, either on blood flow or the healing of damaged tissues in your body. Doctors agree that rubbing on liniment is never a valid alternative to performing a warm-up routine before exercise.

## NICOTINE

Chewing tobacco or smoking cigarettes, a pipe, or cigars is addictive and undermines your health and fitness. Inhaling tobacco smoke introduces nicotine, carbon monoxide, and many toxic chemicals into your bloodstream. Although nicotine causes an increase in your heart rate, it also reduces the flow of blood through your muscles. Carbon monoxide from smoking reduces the available oxygen carried around the body, which in turn reduces your capacity for exercise. The effects of the nicotine you get from smoking a cigarette wear off quickly in terms of athletic performance, but it takes at least 24 hours to clear the carbon monoxide from your blood.

Tobacco use also increases your risk of lung cancer and other cancers, chronic bronchitis, emphysema, heart disease, and circulation disorders. Quitting smoking is the single most important way you can improve your health. Weight control, physical activity, and control of hypertension are also important.

**Effects of smoking**
*Nicotine speeds up your heart rate but it also reduces blood flow through the muscles.*

## PAINKILLERS

The painkillers used today include strong painkillers, known as narcotic analgesics; weak painkillers, such as aspirin and acetaminophen; and local anesthetics, sometimes administered as an injection or in an ointment, cream, or spray.

Strong painkillers such as codeine and morphine are prohibited for use in competitive sports to prevent an individual who has a painful injury from participating. If the pain is partially masked by the use of such painkillers, your perception of pain is dulled by the narcotics, and you imagine it is safe to play. But you run the risk of aggravating the injury or even of causing permanent damage. Taking a narcotic painkiller regularly is also likely to cause addiction.

Weaker painkillers are not prohibited in sports but you should apply the same principles to their use. If an injury is still painful, then it is not safe for you to resume any sport or exercise for which you need to use the injured part.

Occasionally, a doctor gives an injection of a local anesthetic to a professional athlete to deaden the pain of an injury temporarily so that he or she can take part in competition. As with codeine and morphine, such use of painkillers carries a serious risk of aggravating the injury and causing permanent damage.

During televised sports events, you may observe a trainer applying a local anesthetic spray to the injury of a player who is in a lot of pain. The spray acts rapidly but wears off within a few seconds. In your backyard, the application of ice or a sponge or cloth soaked in cold water has a similar effect.

## SLEEPING PILLS

Drugs taken to help you sleep are likely to affect your performance the next morning by interfering with your coordination and concentration. If your doctor has prescribed sleeping pills, and you're in the habit of scheduling your exercise early in the morning, ask your doctor to prescribe a medication that wears off quickly to minimize this hangover effect. However, it's best to avoid sleeping pills altogether.

Some sports authorities prohibit the use of all sedative drugs, including sleeping pills. If you plan to enter a competition, you should not take a sleeping pill within 24 hours of the urine testing.

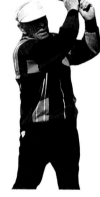

**Sedatives**
*Taking a sleeping pill the night before a workout may affect your coordination and concentration the next day. Hearty daily exercise and a cup of warm milk at bedtime are safer methods of promoting sleep.*

## STIMULANTS

This term includes a wide variety of drugs that range in strength from powerful AMPHETAMINES (see page 136) to weak stimulants such as CAFFEINE (see page 137) and the decongestants used in COLD AND COUGH and HAY-FEVER REMEDIES (see pages 137 and 138). All stimulants are prohibited from use in athletic competitions to prevent athletes from abusing them as a method of masking fatigue or enhancing aggression.

# INDEX OF SPORTS INJURIES

This is a selected list of injuries that may occur during exercise or sports.
Terms in *italics* refer to other terms listed in this A-Z section.
See also references to First Aid in the index of this volume on pages 142 to 144.
For most minor injuries see "RICE" – Rest, Ice, Compression, and Elevation – on page 122.

## A

**Achilles tendinitis**
Inflammation of the tendon that runs from the end of the calf muscle to the back of the ankle, caused either by overuse of the muscles of the lower leg or by friction from a heel counter on the back of a running shoe.

**Arthritis, post-traumatic**
Inflammation of a joint, caused by repeated minor injuries or by a serious injury that has damaged the inside surfaces of the joint.

## B

**Baseball pitchers' elbow**
Pain on the inside or back of the elbow, caused by the stress placed on this joint during pitching.

**Baseball finger**
Injury to the finger, caused by a heavy blow to the tip of the finger. You may not be able to straighten the finger completely, but your doctor may straighten it for you.

**Black eye**
Bruising around the eye, caused by bleeding under the loose skin from a blow to the eye or nose.

**Bowlers' back**
A sharp pain in the back, usually brought on by the twisting action you use when you bowl.

**Boxers' arm**
Pain just above the elbow, caused by repeated punching movements.

**Bursitis**
Inflammation of a bursa, one of the fluid-filled sacs that is found around joints, between or under tendons, and over bony prominences. Each bursa acts as a cushion to reduce friction on the joints.

## C

**Capsulitis**
Inflammation of the lining of a joint, caused by twisting or jarring. This causes stiffness.

**Cauliflower ear**
Deformity of the ear, caused by repeated injury or by a severe blow.

**Charley horse**
Soreness, usually in the thigh muscles, from overstrain or a direct blow.

**Chondromalacia patellae**
A painful softening of the cartilage behind the kneecap that occurs in bicyclists.

**Compartmental syndrome**
Pain in a group of muscles during exercise, which occurs when muscles swell excessively but are confined by the adjoining tissues.

**Concussion**
Headache, possible loss of consciousness, dizziness, blurred vision, nausea, vomiting, and difficulty concentrating that are caused by a blow to the head.

**Cramp**
Painful spasm of a muscle, often in a limb, usually brought on by vigorous exercise.

## D

**Dancers' heel**
See *jumpers' heel*.

**Dead leg**
Temporary loss of sensation in the thigh, usually caused by a direct blow.

**Dislocation**
Displacement of the bones that meet at a joint so that they are temporarily out of their normal positions.

## E

**Epicondylitis**
Painful inflammation of one of the bony prominent areas that lie on either side of the elbow, caused by overuse of the forearm muscles. This commonly occurs in baseball players and tennis players.

## F

**Finger split**
A split in the skin of the hand, caused by overuse or by a faulty grip in sports such as golf, squash, or hockey.

**Flatfoot pain**
Pain on the inside of the ankle, generally caused by a flat-footed running style. See also *Shin splints*.

**Fosbury flop ankle**
Damage to the ankle joint in high-jumpers, caused by rotation of the lower leg on the foot during "takeoff."

**Fracture**
A broken bone, often the result of a direct blow or of falling awkwardly.

**Friction burn**
See *mat burn*.

**Frozen shoulder**
A painful inflammation of the tissue surrounding a shoulder joint, which causes severe limitation of shoulder movements.

## G

**Golfers' elbow**
A painful inflammation on the inside of the elbow, caused by overuse of the muscles in the arm that pull back the hand and wrist. It is commonly caused by poor technique during a golf swing.

**Grass burn**
See *mat burn*.

**Gymnasts' back**
Pain in the back, caused by exercises in which you arch your back and overstretch the muscles and ligaments.

## H

**Handstanders' wrist**
Pain in the back of the wrist when it is moved backward.

**Heat exhaustion**
A condition in which you become dizzy, nauseated, and overtired from exercising too strenuously in hot weather. If untreated, heat exhaustion can lead to heat stroke, which can be fatal (see also page 83).

**Hematoma**
A collection of blood inside your body caused by an injury that damages a blood vessel and results in bleeding.

**Hernia, inguinal**
A condition in which part of the intestine or mesentery (connecting tissue) bulges into the groin or scrotum through a weakness in the muscle wall of the abdomen. It is common in weight lifters.

**Hyperextended elbow**
Pain and instability in the elbow, caused by repeated overstraightening of the elbow.

## J

**Joggers' nipple**
Painful inflammation of the nipples, caused by repeated rubbing against clothes during long-distance running.

**Jumpers' heel**
Pain in your foot on either side of the Achilles tendon, caused when the heel bone jars against the bottom of the shin bone because of poor jumping technique.

**Jumpers' knee**
Painful inflammation of the tendon that attaches the kneecap to the top of the shin bone. This injury is usually caused by repeatedly overstraightening the knee.

# L

**Little leaguers' elbow**
*Baseball pitchers' elbow* in children, which is caused by stress to the elbow from repeatedly attempting to put too much spin on a ball, resulting in the pulling off of a small fragment of bone. Children are now advised to limit their pitching to every third day to prevent this injury, which could interfere with their bone growth.

**Loose body**
A fragment of bone or cartilage that has chipped off a surface inside a joint. If the loose body becomes lodged between the ends of two bones, the joint can temporarily lock in one position.

# M

**Mallet finger**
A painful, bruised, swollen, and bent fingertip joint, often caused by poor technique in catching a baseball.

**March fracture**
A fracture of one of the small bones in the foot, caused by repeated jarring during long-distance walking and marching, running a marathon, or aerobic dancing.

**Mat burn**
Painful abrasion of the skin, caused by a sliding fall on a hard, dry surface or a synthetic surface.

**Metatarsalgia**
Pain in the ball of the foot, caused by damage to the underlying protective tissue pad between the bones and skin. It often results from exercising on hard surfaces in shoes that don't provide adequate support.

**Muscle tear**
Damage caused by overstretching or by a direct blow while a muscle is actively contracting.

# O

**Osgood-Schlatter disease**
Painful inflammation of the bony prominence at the upper end of the shin bone and the adjoining cartilage. It is common in teenagers and normally subsides when the bone stops growing.

# P

**Paddlers' wrist**
Inflammation of the tendons on the outside of the wrist, caused by repeatedly rolling the wrist while you grip the handle of an oar.

**Periostitis**
Painful inflammation of the outer surface of a bone, usually as the result of a blow.

**Pitchers' elbow**
See *baseball pitchers' elbow.*

**Plantar fasciitis**
Inflammation of the tissues in the sole of the foot, causing a painful, tender area in front of the heel; the tenderness is made worse by pressure.

# R

**Riders' strain**
A partial tear of the muscles high in the groin, caused by repeated overstretching. This injury occurs in bicyclists or long-distance runners.

**Rotator cuff tendinitis**
Painful inflammation of the rotator cuff – a structure around the shoulder joint capsule composed of intermingled muscle and tendon fibers.

**Runners' heel**
Pain over the back of the heel, caused by inflammation.

**Runners' knee**
Pain on the outside of the knee, caused by a strain in the fibrous tissue that supports the outside of the knee joint. It occurs in long-distance runners. Inflammation of the tendon of the kneecap (patella) is also called runners' knee.

**Runners' toe**
Painful bleeding under the toenail, caused by damage to the nail bed. It arises from a direct blow or from pressure caused by tight running shoes.

# S

**Shin splints**
Pain in the front and sides of the lower leg that is caused by exercise and relieved by rest. Shin splints is a catchall term applied to leg pain from tendon or muscle strain, a *compartmental syndrome,* or a *stress fracture.*

**Shot-putters' finger**
Painful inflammation of the tissues on the sides of the first three fingers of the hand, often caused by stress from accelerating the throw of the shot.

**Skaters' heel**
Inflammation of the bursa (fluid-filled sac) that cushions the heel bone, caused by friction from wearing skates that are too tight.

**Soccer ankle**
Painful, stiff ankle, usually resulting from repeated kicks to the ankle or minor ligament sprains.

**Spondylolisthesis**
Back pain sometimes caused by one vertebra slipping over the one below it.

**Sprain**
A slight tear in a ligament or in the capsule lining a joint, usually caused by an injury that forces the joint beyond its normal range of movement.

**Squash players' finger**
Pain in the back of the hand, caused by gripping the racket too tightly with the thumb and index finger.

**Strain**
A tear in a muscle or tendon, or a stretched muscle that hurts, usually caused by an injury that forces the muscle beyond its normal range of movement. A strain is difficult to distinguish from a *sprain;* both are common injuries.

**Stress fracture**
A break in a bone that occurs as a result of repeated jarring, rather than a sudden violent blow. The most common sites for a stress fracture are the foot or shin in a long-distance walker or runner, and the wrist in a gymnast.

**Supraspinatus tendinitis**
Inflammation of one of the tendons in the shoulder, causing pain as the arm is moved in an arc between 60 and 120 degrees vertically away from the body.

**Surfers' nodules**
Bony swellings on the front of the shin bones and top of the foot, formed by repeatedly knocking the foot or leg against a surfboard.

**Swimmers' shoulder**
Painful inflammation of the soft tissues around the shoulder, a form of *rotator cuff tendinitis* caused by repeatedly doing swimming strokes that require you to extend your arm outward – for example, while doing the backstroke.

# T

**Tear**
See *strain.*

**Tendinitis**
Painful inflammation of a tendon, caused by repeated movement or prolonged pressure. The pain becomes more intense when you move or squeeze the tendon.

**Tennis elbow**
Painful inflammation on the outside of the elbow, caused by overuse of the muscles of the forearm. Other racket sports and activities may also be a cause.

**Tenosynovitis**
Inflammation of the lining of a tendon, usually caused by friction from repeated movement of the affected part of the body. In addition to pain and swelling, there is often a crackling sensation when the tendon is moved. Tenosynovitis of the wrist is common in baseball and basketball.

**Throwers' elbow**
See *baseball pitchers' elbow.*

**Triple jumpers' heel**
See *plantar fasciitis.*

**Turf toe**
See *runners' toe.*

# W

**Wrestlers' or boxers' ear**
See *cauliflower ear.*

# INDEX

Page numbers in *italics* refer to illustrations and captions.

## A

abdominal injuries 96-97
abdominal muscles, stretching exercises for *24-25*
abdominal muscle strain *86*
abdominal pain 97
acetyl coenzyme A 23
Achilles tendon injuries 112, 140
Achilles tendon protector *78*
adductor muscle strain 113, 114
adenosine triphosphate 23
aerobic chemical processes 22-23
aerobic dancing 21
    at home *28*
    shoes for *79*
aerobic exercise 20-23, 64-65
    burning fat through 23, *35*
    after injury 121
    during pregnancy 44
aging and exercise 45-47
alcohol 36, 136
    hypothermia and 70, 136
    increased risk of injuries after use of 70, 72, 73
amenorrhea 83
amino acid supplements 37
amphetamines 136
anabolic steroids 138
    use of by children 41
anaerobic chemical processes 23
anaerobic exercise 23, *27, 35*
anemia 53-54
angina 51, 95
ankle injuries 109
    rehabilitation exercises after 125
    see also Fosbury flop ankle; soccer ankle
antibiotics 136
antihistamines 136
anti-inflammatory drugs 99, *119*, 120, 136-137
anxiety, relief from 19
arch supports 77
arm injuries 95, 98-107
    see also boxers' arm
arm swings *46*
arthritis 51
    post-traumatic 140
arthroscope 111
aspirin *119*, 120, 136-137
assessment of fitness level 60-61
assisted exercise 120
    swimming as a form of *121*
asthma 53
    drugs for 137
athletic supporter *81*
ATP (adenosine triphosphate) 23

## B

back injuries 90-93
    see also bowlers' back; gymnasts' back
back pain *86*, 92
    benefits of exercise for 50
    case history 133
    disc problems causing 50, 91, 92
    jogging and 50
    rehabilitation exercises for 131-132
    swimming and 50
back strain 90
balanced diet 34-37

baseball finger *71*, 107, 140
baseball injuries *86*, 102
baseball pitchers' elbow *104*, 140
basketball *106*, 109
beta blockers 51, 137
biceps strain 100
bicycle helmets 80, *80*, 89
bicycle riding see cycling
bill of rights for young athletes 40
black eye 140
blister *107*
blood cholesterol 19, 36
blood doping 137
blood pressure
    high 51
    isometric exercises and 27
blood sugar levels during exercise 52, 54
blow
    to abdomen 96-97
    to head 88-89
    to solar plexus 96-97
body, effect of exercise on 14-17
body bends *46*
bowlers' back 140
boxers' arm 140
brain damage 88
bras 77, 94
breast injuries 94
    see also joggers' nipple
bruises 122
bruising to coccyx 92
bursitis 140
    in elbow 103
    in hip 113
    in knee 110
    in shoulder *86*, 99
buttock strain 113

## C

caffeine 36, 137
calf injuries 112
cancer prevention 19
capsulitis 140
carbohydrates 34-35
cardiac output 16
cardiopulmonary resuscitation 89
cardiovascular fitness 14-15, 16, 61, *68*
carpal tunnel syndrome 105
cartilage injuries 110-111
cast, plaster *106, 120, 124*
cauliflower ear 140
cervical strain 91
charley horse 140
checkup before starting exercise program 68, 72, 73
chemical processes 22-23
chest injuries 94-95
chest pain 95
childbirth, exercising after *45*
children 40-42
    bill of rights for young athletes 40
    elbow injuries in 102
    use of anabolic steroids by 41
cholesterol 19, 36
chondromalacia patellae 110, 140
cigarette-smoking 19, 139
circuit training *29*
clothing for exercise 52, 76-77, 94
cocaine 137
coccyx injuries 92
codeine 137, 138
cold and cough remedies 137
collarbone fracture *86*
Colles fracture 106
compartmental syndrome 140
compression bandages 122
concussion 88-89, 140

conditioning 64
consciousness, loss of, first aid for 89
contact sports 88, *105*
cooling down 24, 75
coronary heart disease 12, *19*, 40-41, *42, 51*
corticosteroid drugs 105, *119*, 138
"couch potato" *40*
    case history 42
cough remedies 137
CPR (cardiopulmonary resuscitation) 89
cramp *119*, 140
cross-country skiing *30*
cycling
    helmet for 80, *80*, 89
    when overweight 49

## D

dancers' heel 140
danger signals 51, 69, 72, *73*, 82, 97, 124
dead leg 140
dehydration, preventing 36-37, 43
depression, relief from 19
diabetes, benefits of exercise for 52
diarrhea remedies 138
diarrhea, runners' 83
diet, balanced 34-37
    weight reduction and 48
dieting medications 138
digestive system, effect of exercise on *14, 15*
disc, prolapsed *86*, 91
    case history 133
dislocation 140
    elbow 102
    finger *86*, 107
    hip 113
    kneecap 110
    shoulder 99, 100, 101
diuretics 138
drug abuse 136, 137
drugs 136-139
    increased risk of injuries after use of 70, 72, 73
    use of after injury 120
    see also individual drugs and groups of drugs by name
dynamic muscle exercises 26-27

## E

eating, timing of exercise and 35
elastic support hose 52
elbow guards 103
elbow injuries 102-104
    see also baseball pitchers' elbow; epicondylitis; golfers' elbow; hyperextended elbow; little leaguers' elbow; tennis elbow
elbow pain, case history 127
elevation of injuries 122
endurance 59
    self-assessment 60
epicondylitis 140
epilepsy 54
equipment 76-81
    protective 72, 73, 80-81
    research on 76
exercise
    benefits of 11-13, 18-19, 40-49, 50-52, 63
    daily 13, *65*
    effects of, on body 14-17
    at home 28-29
    after injury see rehabilitation exercises

    life expectancy and 13, 63
    need for 10-13
    problems of excess 82, *82*
    safety during 66-83
    social activity and 30
    types of 20-21, 24-27, 30
exercise diary 65
exercise machines 64, *121*
    isokinetic *118*
    stair-climbing 21
    use of, in health clubs 32-33
    use of, at home 28-29
exercise mat 21, *28*
exercise stress test 68
eye injuries 80, 81
    see also black eye

## F

fainting during exercise 69, 72
falls and collisions 95
fat stores and aerobic exercise 17, 34, *35*
femur, fracture of 113, 114
fibula, fracture of 112
finger injuries *86*, 106-107
    see also baseball finger; finger split; mallet finger; shot-putters' finger; squash players' finger
fingernail hematoma *107*
finger split 140
first aid
    for loss of consciousness 89
    for neck injuries 93
    "RICE" routine of 117, 122-123, 127
fitness 56-65
    elements of 58-59
    level of, how to improve 64-65
    self-assessment 45, 60-61
flatfoot pain 140
flexibility 59, 64
    exercises for 24-25
    self-assessment 60
flexor tendinitis 107
fluid intake 36-37
food and exercise see diet, balanced
football 80, 81, *114*
foot injuries *86*, 108-109
    see also metatarsalgia
footwear see shoes
forearm injuries *86*, 102-106
Fosbury flop ankle 140
fracture 140
    ankle 140
    arm 102, 103
    collarbone *86*
    Colles 106
    elbow *104*
    of femur 113, 114
    of fibula 112
    finger 107
    foot *86*
    forearm *86*, 102, 106
    of humerus *86*, 100
    leg 112
    march 141
    of olecranon 103
    of radius *86*, 102, 106
    rib 94-95
    of scaphoid *106*
    shoulder 99
    skull 88
    stress 112, 141
    of tibia 112
    toe *86*
    wrist 106
friction burn 140
frozen shoulder 140

## G

glycogen *17, 22, 34*
goggles 80, 81, *86*
golf *30*
golfers' elbow *71, 86, 104,* 140
grass burn 140
groin injuries *86,* 113, 134
    case history 115
    see also riders' strain
groin pain, case history 115
growth hormone 138
Guillain-Barré syndrome, case
   history 55
gymnastics injuries *87,* 106
gymnasts' back 140

## H

hamstring
    injury, rehabilitation exercises
      after 135
    strain 114
    stretching exercise for *24, 75,*
      135
hand injuries 106-107
handstanders' wrist 140
hay-fever remedies 136, 138
head injuries 88-89
health clubs 32-33, *47*
heart
    effect of exercise on *14-15,* 16
    testing efficiency of 61, *68*
heart attack 95
    exercising after 51
    warning signs of 51, 69, 72, 73
heart disease   see coronary heart
   disease
heart failure, benefits of exercise
   for 51
heart rate 16, 61
heat exhaustion 83, 140
heat treatment *120,* 121, 123
heel counter *78*
heel pain 108
    see also dancers' heel; jumpers'
      heel; runners' heel; skaters'
      heel
heel spur 108
helmets 80, *80,* 81, 89
hematoma 140
    in an abdominal muscle 96
    after a head injury 88
    fingernail *107*
hematuria, runners' 83
hemorrhage, brain 88
hernia, inguinal 113, 134, 140
    case history 115
high blood pressure 51
hip injuries 113
hockey, ice *105, 122*
hormones 138
human body, overview of *14-15,*
   *86-87*
humerus, fracture of *86,* 100
hydrotherapy 118, *119,* 120
hyperextended elbow *103,* 140
hypertension 51
hypoglycemia 52, 54

## I

ibuprofen 120, 136-137
ice hockey *105,* 122
ice packs 120, 122, 123
illness, chronic   see medical
   disorders
infections 54, 72-73
    following head injury 88
inflammation 122, 123
    bone   see periostitis

bowel 83
bursa   see bursitis
elbow   see tennis elbow
foot 108
joint   see arthritis, post-
   traumatic
knee   see runners' knee
leg   see Osgood-Schlatter
   disease
nipple   see joggers' nipple
reduction of *119*
tendon   see tendinitis;
   tenosynovitis
inguinal hernia   113, 134, 140
    case history 115
injuries 85-115, 122, 140-141
    adapting to 121
    in children *41*
    common sites of 86-87
    internal 97
    poor technique as cause of 71,
      *72, 73, 103,* 127
    recent 69, *72, 73*
    rehabilitation after 70, 117-135
    shoes and *72, 73, 78,* 109, 112
    see also specific injuries
insoles *78*
insomnia, prevention of 19
internal injuries and damage 97
iron supplements 37
isokinetic exercises 26, 118
isometric exercises 26, 27
isotonic exercises 26

## J

jewelry 29, 76
jockstrap *81*
joggers' nipple 94, 140
jogging 20, 49
    back pain and 50
    cooling down after 75
    warming up before 74
    see also running
joint injuries   see arthritis, post-
   traumatic; capsulitis
jumpers' heel 140
jumpers' knee 141
jumping rope 29

## K

kidney rupture 96
knee injuries  *69, 87,* 110-111
    rehabilitation exercises after
      129-130
    surgery for 111
    see also chondromalacia
      patellae; jumpers' knee;
      runners' knee
Krebs cycle *23*

## L

lactic acid *22, 27*
leg injuries 112
    see also ankle injuries; knee
      injuries
leg lifts *124*
life expectancy 13, 63
ligament injuries 106
    ankle 109
    finger 106
    foot 109
    hand 106
    knee *69,* 110, 111
    wrist 105
limb injuries 98-115
liniments 75, 139
liquid intake 36-37
little leaguers' elbow *86,* 141

liver rupture 96
longshoremen and physical
   energy expenditure 11
loose body 102, 141
low-impact aerobics 21
low-intensity exercise 48-49
lumbar puncture *55*
lung, perforated 94
lungs
    effect of exercise on 14, 15, 16
    injuries to 94-95

## M

mallet finger 107, 141
mall walking 63
march fracture 141
marijuana 136
massage 75, 118, *119*
mat burn 141
maximum oxygen consumption
   test 16, 60
medical disorders
    benefits and dangers of
      exercise in relation to 50-54
    choice of exercise and 50, *72, 73*
medication   see drugs
meniscectomy 111
menstrual cycle 19, 41, *83*
metatarsalgia 141
minerals 37
mitochondria *17, 23*
mobility exercises 132
motivation *12, 30*
mouth guard 80
muscle injuries 94, 95, 97
    abdominal 96
    arm 100, 103
    calf 112
    chest 94
    knee 110
    leg 112
    recovery from 82
    shoulder 98-99
    thigh 114
    see also strain
muscle pain *22*
muscles
    effect of exercise on *14, 15, 17,*
      34
    increase in bulk of *26,* 27
    metabolism and 22-23
muscle weakness, case history 55
myoglobin *17*

## N

neck injuries 90-91
    first aid for 93
nerve damage 100
nicotine 139
"no hands" squat *75*
nonsteroidal anti-inflammatory
   drugs (NSAIDs) 99, *119,* 120, 136-
   137
nutritional products and
   supplements 36-37

## O

obesity 18, 40, 48-49
older people and exercise 45-46
olecranon, fracture of 103
orthotic appliances 77
Osgood-Schlatter disease 141
osteoarthritis 110
osteoporosis 18
overexercising 41, *72, 73,* 82-83
overweight 18, 40, 48-49
overweight teenager, case history
   42

## P

paddlers' wrist 141
pain 122
    ignoring 123
    in parts of body   see part of
      body involved, e.g., back pain
    referred 113
painkillers 139
Parkinson's disease 53
passivity, avoiding *13*
pectoral muscle strain 94, 95
pelvic floor exercises *44*
periostitis 141
peripheral vascular disease,
   benefits of exercise for 52
perspiration 36, 37
physical activity   see exercise
"pins-and-needles" sensation 104
plantar fasciitis 108, 141
plaster cast *106, 120,* 124
popliteal muscle strain 110
postnatal exercises 45
posture 18
    flexibility exercises and 24
pre-aerobic activities 48-49
pregnancy and exercise 43-44
prolapsed disc *86,* 91
    case history 133
protective equipment *72, 73,* 80-81
protein 35-36
pulse 16
    resting 61
pulse recovery time 61

## Q

quadriceps
    muscle strain 114
    rehabilitation exercises for 129
    stretching exercise for *25*

## R

race walking *62*
racquetball
    goggles for *80,* 81
    injuries *86*
radius *103*
    fracture of *86, 102,* 106
recovery process 122-123
referred pain 113
rehabilitation after injury 117-135
rehabilitation exercises 121, 123,
   124-135
    after ankle sprain 125
    for back pain 131-132
    after groin injury 134
    after hamstring injury 135
    after knee injuries 129-130
    after shoulder injuries 128-129
    for tennis elbow 126
rehabilitation program 121
relaxation exercises 29
rest after injury 122
resting pulse 61
resuscitation, cardiopulmonary 89
retirement, case history 47
rib injuries 94-95
"RICE" routine of first aid 117, 122-
   123, 127
riders' strain 141
rotator cuff injuries 98, *99*
rotator cuff tendinitis *86,* 141
    see also swimmers' shoulder
rowing *100*
runners' diarrhea 83
runners' heel 141
runners' hematuria 83
runners' knee 110, 141
runners' toe 141

running 70, 110, 112
    avoiding injury when 70
    choice of shoes for 70, 78-79
    see also jogging
rupture
    Achilles tendon 112
    disc  see disc, prolapsed
    kidney 96
    liver 96
    spleen 94, 96, 97

## S

safety 66-83
    clothing and 77
    equipment 72, 73, 80-81
salt loss 36
sciatica 92
scaphoid, fracture of 106
sedatives 139
shin splints 86, 87, 112, 141
shoes 70, 77-79
    corrective 77
    injuries and 72, 73, 78, 109, 112
    orthotic appliances in 77
    well-designed 78
shot-putters' finger 141
shoulder dislocation 86, 99
    case history 101
shoulder immobilizer 101
shoulder injuries 86, 95, 98-100
    case history 101
    rehabilitation exercises after
        128-129
    see also frozen shoulder;
        shoulder dislocation;
        supraspinatus tendinitis;
        swimmers' shoulder
shoulder rolls 46
shoulders, stretching exercises for
    24, 45, 74, 128
sit-ups 60
skaters' heel 141
skiing 69
    cross-country 30
skiing injuries 87, 107
skull fracture 88
sleep 19

sleeping pills 139
smoking 19, 139
soccer ankle 141
spine injuries 90-93
spleen rupture 94, 96, 97
spondylolisthesis 86, 141
sports and exercises
        popularity ratings of 31
        see also individual sports and
            exercises by name
sprain 92, 141
    ankle 109
    hip 113
    knee 69
    rib 94
    treatment for 119
    wrist 105
squash injuries 86
squash players' finger 141
stair-climbing 13, 21, 65
steroids, anabolic 138
    use of by children 41
stiffness, muscle 82
stimulants 139
"stinger" 100
stitch 97
strain 92, 141
    abdominal muscle 86
    adductor muscle 113, 114
    back 90
    biceps 100
    buttock 113
    cervical 91
    chest muscle 94
    groin 86, 115
    hamstring 114
    knee ligament 110
    popliteal muscle 110
    quadriceps muscle 114
    rib 94
    riders' 141
    rotator cuff 99
    shoulder 98
    treatment for 119
    triceps 103
strapping 81, 119
strength 59
        self-assessment 60

strength exercises 26-27, 32-33, 64
    after childbirth 45
stress fracture 112, 141
stress test 68
stretching exercises 24-25, 64
    after childbirth 45
    after injury 118, 121, 125, 126
        128, 131, 135
    during pregnancy 44
    warming up with 46, 74-75
stroke, benefits of exercise after 52
stroke volume 16
supplements, nutritional 36, 37
supraspinatus tendinitis 141
surfers' nodules 141
surgery 98, 111, 118
    case histories 101, 115, 118
swimmers' shoulder 87, 98, 141
swimming
        for exercising shoulder
            injuries 128
        when overweight 48, 49
        relief of back pain through 50
        during pregnancy 43-44
        as therapy 87, 12
swimming injuries 87
synovitis 99, 111

## T

taping 81, 119
tear  see strain
tendinitis 107, 141
    Achilles 112, 140
    flexor 107
    rotator cuff 86, 141
    supraspinatus 141
tendon injuries to hand 107
tennis 58, 65, 79
tennis elbow 71, 103, 104, 141
    case history 127
    rehabilitation exercises for 126
tenosynovitis 105, 141
thigh injuries 114
    see also charley horse; dead leg
thighs, stretching exercises for 25,
    75
tibia, fracture of 112

tobacco, nicotine and 139
toe injuries 86
    see also runners' toe
track and field sports injuries 87
treatment for exercise injuries
    111, 118-123, 136-139
triceps pain 100
triceps strain 103
triple jumpers' heel   141

## U

ulna 102
unconsciousness 52, 89
upper arm injuries 86, 100

## V

varicose veins 52
viral infection, "no exercise"
    rule for 54
vitamins and minerals 37
VO$_2$ max test 16, 60

## W

walking 11, 13, 20, 62-63, 65
    choice of shoes for 79
    when overweight 49
    during pregnancy 43-44
warming up 24, 46, 72, 73, 74-75
warnings  see danger signals
water sports and safety 81
weight-lifting 27, 35, 138
weight reduction 18, 48-49
weights
    ankle 125, 129, 130, 135
    small 26, 27, 62, 126, 129
weight training 26-27
whiplash 91
wrestling 95
wrist injuries 105-106
    see also handstanders' wrist;
        paddlers' wrist

## Y

yoga 25

**Photograph sources:**
Ace Photo Agency **69** (top left); **69**
    (right)
Action Images **138** (center)
Action-Plus **97** (bottom left); **102** (top);
    **103** (bottom right); **104** (center)
Allsport (UK) Ltd **97** (bottom right);
    **100** (bottom right); **103** (top); **109**
    (bottom right); **111** (bottom left)
Art Directors' Photo Library **138** (top)
Colorsport **41** (top right); **41** (center
    right); **89** (bottom right); **89** (bottom
    right); **95** (center); **95** (bottom); **114**
    (bottom)
Mary Evans Picture Library **10** (top
    right)
Leslie Howling **43** (bottom left)
The Image Bank **7** (top); **9** (center); **10**
    (bottom left); **11** (center); **30** (top
    right); **30** (center right); **30** (bottom
    left); **30** (bottom right); **39** (center);
    **53** (center); **54** (bottom right); **57**
    (center); **70** (right); **71** (top left); **71**
    (bottom left); **76** (center); **76** (bottom
    right); **77** (center left); **83** (center); **85**
    (center); **93** (top right); **93** (bottom
    left); **98** (bottom left); **120** (top); **123**
    (center left); **136** (bottom)

Impact **103** (top right); **137** (top)
National Medical Slide Bank (UK) **41**
    (center); **102** (center); **106** (top right); **107**
    (center left); **119** (bottom right)
The Photographers' Library **67** (center)
Pictor International **13** (top right)
Science Photo Library **2** (top right); **2**
    (bottom left); **17** (top right); **17** (bottom
    right); **17** (left); **17** (bottom left); **35**
    (bottom right); **104** (bottom left); **109**
    (center right); **111** (insert)
Sporting Pictures (UK) Ltd **106** (bottom
    left)
Tony Stone Worldwide **2** (top left); **12**
    (bottom right); **41** (bottom left); **50** (bot-
    tom left); **53** (bottom left); **70** (center); **75**
    (bottom right); **102** (bottom left); **105**
    (bottom left); **122** (center); **123** (center);
    and **front cover**
John Watney **107** (center right)
Dr Robert Youngson **111** (center right)
Zefa Picture Library **11** (top left); **13** (top
    left); **21** (bottom right); **22** (bottom left);
    **76** (top left); **77** (center); **107** (center); **122**
    (top); **123** (bottom right)
**All sports clothes and equipment courtesy
of Lillywhites, Piccadilly Circus, London**

**Commissioned
photography:**
Jim Forest
Susanna Price
Clive Streeter

**Airbrushing:**
Paul Desmond
Janos Marffy

**Retouching:**
Roy Flooks

**Illustrators:**
Russell Barnet
Paul Desmond
David Fathers
Tony Graham
Andrew Green
Marks Illustration
    and Design
Lydia Umney
Philip Wilson
John Woodcock

**Index:** Susan Bosanko

Reader's Digest Fund for the Blind is
publisher of the Large-Type Edition of
*Reader's Digest.* For subscription information about this magazine, please
contact Reader's Digest Fund for the
Blind, Inc., Dept. 250, Pleasantville, N.Y.
10570.

**"Young Athlete's Bill of Rights,"** page 40,
**reproduced with permission of American
Medical Association** (*AJDC*, Feb 1988)